Spotlight on General Practice

Preparing for the demands of clinical governance and revalidation

Sally Irvine

and

Hilary Haman

Foreword by

Professor Mike Pringle

Chairman of Council, Royal College of General Practitioners

RADCLIFFE MEDICAL PRESS

Radcliffe Medical Press Ltd
18 Marcham Road, Abingdon, Oxon OX14 1AA

British Library Cataloguing in Publication Data
A catalogue record for this book is available from the British Library.

ISBN 1 85775 496 4

Typeset by Aarontype Ltd, Easton, Bristol
Printed and bound by TJ International Ltd, Padstow, Cornwall

Contents

Foreword

General practice presents a complex environment in which to work. In a medium-sized practice there will be at least 10 doctors, nurses and managers. That involves 45 one-to-one relationships and then a number of group relationships. The practice itself will have shared values, a culture, and a self-image that it presents to patients and the rest of the health service.

The external environment has also become increasingly complex. A practice cannot survive by hiding away and getting on with clinical care. Each is part of a primary care organisation and each has key relationships with health authorities and community and secondary care trusts.

And external bodies are increasingly interested in what happens inside practices. The rise in accountability – of individual doctors and nurses and of practices – through clinical audit, quality indicators, costs, revalidation and health needs assessment has been startling. If we were ever able to say 'trust me, I'm a general practitioner' that is definitely no longer the reality today.

Just as it is almost a surprise to observe the high quality of most primary care in such a complex world, it is not surprising that practices can be dysfunctional in either their internal or external relationships. Sally Irvine and Hilary Haman are the acknowledged experts in diagnosing and addressing dysfunction in general practice. They have been visiting and analysing practices for many years and they bring all their experience to bear on this remarkable book.

Good practices do not happen by serendipity. They have shared values and sound relationships. They have good

management systems and internal accountability. They understand their place in, and contribution to, the wider health
service. They have a sense of community. This book is the bible
for understanding these issues and building a modern practice.

Professor Mike Pringle
Chairman of Council
Royal College of General Practitioners
August 2000

About the authors

Sally Irvine was made an Honorary Fellow of the RCGP in 1995, a Fellow of the Association of Managers in General Practice (AMGP) in the same year and is a Member of the Institute of Healthcare Management.

She has over 18 years' experience of working in and with many aspects of healthcare delivery. She was the General Administrator of the RCGP from 1984–94, and was President of the AMGP from 1990–94. She chaired Newcastle City Health NHS Trust from its inception in 1993 to 1999. It was a Trust that delivered community, mental health and rehabilitative care in the north east of England. Currently she is appointed a lay member of the General Dental Council and a hospital manager under the Mental Health Act. Her most recent appointments are as an Arbitration and Conciliation Advisory Service (ACAS) Arbitrator, a member of the Newcastle Common Purpose Advisory Board and a Trustee of Total Learning Challenge.

In recent years Sally has concentrated on her work as a professional practice consultant in primary care. She has published many texts on organisational and developmental issues within primary care and writes regularly for the professional press.

Hilary Haman is a Fellow of the Chartered Institute of Personnel Development and a Member of the Institute of Healthcare Management.

She has over 20 years' experience in personnel management including the running of human resource departments in both the public and private sectors. Hilary first became professionally involved in primary healthcare in 1986 when she joined the RCGP in London as Head of Personnel.

Since 1990 she has worked as an independent management consultant mainly in general practice although she has other clients in the private, public and voluntary sectors. Her work encompasses providing advice on personnel issues, including the application of employment law, designing and running management development courses and, with Sally Irvine as Haman and Irvine Associates, undertaking organisational reviews of individual practices and developing management tools for general practice.

She writes extensively on management and personnel issues within primary care and lives in Cardiff with her husband and son.

Introduction

Healthcare is under scrutiny as never before. The way that health is delivered – who, how, where, at what cost – is changing exponentially. This is in response to many factors, not least the amazing pace of scientific discovery, the revolution in the way people both see their own health needs and regard the professionals who try to meet them, and the response of parliament to these factors. Accountability and performance review have been talked about in various ways for over 20 years and neither the government nor the profession has taken it seriously enough to deliver it, except patchily. Much of such better practice and good intent of the past years is represented by the practices that form the basis of the examples and case studies in this book.

It is now 'high noon'. The seriousness of the government intent to obtain better performance from clinical teams has been demonstrated in the NHS Plan with a firm, centralised approach to monitoring (DoH, 2000). There are two particular developments that will make enormous demands on general practitioners (GPs). The first is managerially led clinical governance and the second is professionally led revalidation of doctors. The clear message is that the activities and leading-edge developments of the enthusiasts are now needed from everyone. It is against this background of governmental determination to assure return on increased investment in the National Health Service (NHS), and these twin developments of clinical governance and revalidation that this book is written. The diagnosis and treatment plans arising from our work with practices and primary care will help those working in this field meet the demands the new world continues to make.

What this book tries to do

There is much greater recognition of the inter-relationship between clinical and organisational management today, that the delivery of high-quality care, in which patients have confidence, is dependent on high-quality clinical skills practised in a safe, efficient and well-managed environment. Indeed, modern developments in general practice, and medicine more widely, are designed to give greater involvement to patients in their own care, and to enhance the accountability of medicine to the public. Foremost among these is clinical governance, together with the changing role of doctors as advocates and commissioners, modern licensing and certification arrangements for all the health professions, and cross-boundary education and learning. All these conspire to increase the need for the clinical/organisational relationship to be developed further.

The authors have a unique perspective on change and development in general practice and primary care, and the lessons for the future that can be drawn from it. Part of that unique perspective lies in the fact that they are lay observers of the medical scene. Not being medically qualified helps them take a more detached and dispassionate view of how general practice delivers patient care, but at the same time gives them great insight into the essential and unique service provided by general practice and family medicine in this country.

In this book they draw on their wide experience of more than 18 years' of visiting and analysing over 200 individual practices and partnerships. The book itself is written for all those involved in the changing primary care scene, healthcare professionals, managers within primary care and those in a wider commissioning scene. It includes the policy and decision makers, commentators and observers of the primary care world, for whom knowledge of how general practice works is vital.

How it is structured

The book concentrates on revealing the key underlying issues that inhibit effective relationships and developments in general practice and consequently will hamper the effective integration of the requirements of clinical governance and revalidation. It relies heavily on illustrating and emphasising these through examples rooted in real life. It starts by looking briefly at the context of modern general practice and today's approach to healthcare. It goes on to describe the process of diagnostic consultancy that forms the backdrop of the authors' experiences and knowledge. Chapters 3–6 then analyse the lessons to be derived from these experiences.

The key issues derived from the past, which will continue to face general practice today and tomorrow, are illustrated not only through the many small examples throughout the book, but also revealed in depth through four extensive case studies in Part 3. These studies are based on actual practices visited, anonymised to retain confidentiality. All those working in primary care will undoubtedly recognise in them some elements of their own experience.

In the final chapter, we reflect on potential future developments in primary care, and how the underlying problems identified and the lessons learnt relate to that future.

Background to diagnostic consultancy in general practice

When Sally Irvine joined the Royal College of General Practitioners (RCGP) in 1983 as its new General Administrator, she was invited to visit and provide managerial comment on the practices of the some of the officers of the College. The result was revealing to them and to her. The impressive clinical care was undoubted. However, it was clear that there was a need for greater understanding of the relationship between that good clinical care and the development of a well-motivated, well-managed team, able to deliver patient and practice services in the most effective and co-ordinated way. The potential for doctors to delegate to others safely and in a way acceptable to them, together with a proper valuing of the contribution made by clinical and non-clinical colleagues, was not fully recognised. Example 1 is from that era.

Example I

Limekiln Surgery was judged to be a fairly advanced surgery in 1983. It had one of the earliest computer systems, ran its surgeries with appointments only and had dedicated treatment rooms run by the practice nurses. However, clinical meetings were dominated by the doctors' agendas, nurses stood outside consulting rooms waiting to hear when the doctor was free to discuss a patient and receptionists were encouraged to see their jobs as protecting doctors, not enabling patients.

Through a process of sensitive information gathering, Sally Irvine was able to combine her experience as a manager and management consultant with knowledge of the workings and pressures of general practice. A unique diagnostic consultancy service for management in general practice was born, which expanded when Hilary Haman joined the College as Personnel Director. Hilary brought with her extensive experience of personnel management, including industrial relations, from both the private and public sectors. Her in-depth knowledge and understanding of employment law and its application to primary care provided practices with sound, pragmatic advice. She and Sally formed a consultancy service offered both through the RCGP and the Association of Managers in General Practice (AMGP).

The demand and need were such that both institutions recognised the value of extending the capacity of their two experts by developing a cadre of consultants across the country that could apply the same techniques and skills. The Practice Consultancy Programme was directed by Sally Irvine and Hilary Haman and funded by the Department of Health (DoH). Over 70 people across a wide range of skills and backgrounds in general practice, the wider health service and health-related areas gained experience and expertise in this unique process. Sally and Hilary continue to provide the service today through their independent consultancy, Haman and Irvine Associates.

The practices

Over 18 years this diagnostic service has been offered in more than 200 practices across the length and breadth of the UK, from the northern isles of Scotland, the Welsh valleys and Northern Ireland to the English industrial heartland and leafy shires. They have ranged from single-handed to 11-partner practices, with and without associates or assistants. Practices have been housed in a wide range of premises from health-authority owned clinics to premises owned by partner consortia. They have been managed in an enormous variety of ways, from partners only, partners and spouses, and senior receptionists to high-flying business managers. They have been training and non-training practices, high-income and low-income, dispensing and non-dispensing.

There have been three main categories of clients. First, most of the practices visited have been self-selected – they have sought this type of help themselves. By and large they already have some insights about the performance of their practice, as well as the will to improve and develop, or to test them in some way against an external benchmark. Indeed, the simple fact of asking external consultants to come into the practice implies a level of self-confidence and awareness that marks them out.

Second, there are practices identified by others as needing help. The need to integrate and improve the educational process in practices across all members of the team was recognised in 1998 (CMO, 1998). Partly as a consequence, some apparently dysfunctional practices have been encouraged by health authorities to seek external help to develop practice plans and developmental opportunities for staff. Example 2 demonstrates this, as does Case Study D in Chapter 10.

Example 2

Cross Health Authority decided to pilot practice and personal development plans in volunteer practices that would not normally be willing or able to fund external support. In the Light Surgery two 'away days' were held with the whole practice team, facilitated by external diagnostic consultants. As a result, a first draft plan for the practice's future was agreed, and individual development plans for individual members of the team were settled. This meant, for instance, that one partner's wish to develop his interest in sports medicine – an issue that had caused much concern and disquiet until then – could be accommodated within his personal development plan, but would not form part of the priorities of the practice.

Third, the nervousness about what primary care groups (PCGs), local health groups (LHGs) in Wales and local healthcare co-operatives (LHCs) in Scotland, and later primary care trusts (PCTs) in England, are going to demand of practices has provoked some practices into seeking external help. In particular this has provided opportunities for the practice to review its priorities and plans for the future, as shown in Example 3.

Example 3

Cardigan Terrace Surgery had six partners and had not managed to get their nominated partner on to the LHG. They were very nervous about being left out, being 'told what to do' by the LHG and not being able to influence it.

They organised a facilitated 'away day' to identify the practice's strengths and weaknesses, and to discuss why they were not involved with the LHG in the way they wanted. The event revealed a number of significant concerns: there were varying degrees of enthusiasm among the partners; concerns about workload and succession within the practice were common; there was a lack of explicit guidelines on clinical care. Above all, the partners faced up to the reputation the practice had locally for being 'a dinosaur'. They spent time discussing those revelations. As a consequence of doing so in a protected environment, the practice felt more cohesive and confident in identifying a LHG role for themselves, how to deliver it and ways of handling developments in the future.

Over the 18 years of visiting practices it has become absolutely clear that the most important issues facing practices do not relate to type or size, or whether they have been fundholding or not, inner city or rural, active in local commissioning or not. The lessons and their consistency appear to relate more to the nature of the work of general practice itself, the educational and training experiences of all those working within primary care, and the attitudes and motivation of the primary healthcare team, particularly the doctors. Variations in style and performance have a great deal to do with individual behaviour and behaviour within groups.

Perhaps for this reason, diagnostic consultancy is tricky. It needs considerable skill, a background of senior managerial responsibility, and knowledge of general practice at both the micro and macro levels. The process requires an ability to think quickly, to be authoritative but not dogmatic, good listening skills and the ability to give encouragement to help the practice face difficult issues. It provides an opportunity for people to think about what they are doing and why, and explain both plainly to others.

This book offers lessons drawn from our peculiar and privileged experience. Those lessons are as relevant to all practices today as they were to the individual practices that benefited directly at the time. We believe that the messages of this book can contribute to the positive development of general practice in the challenging world of 21st century healthcare. They provide effective preparation for the demands of clinical governance and revalidation.

Sally Irvine
sally@sallyirvine.demon.co.uk

Hilary Haman
hhaman@global.co.uk

Part 1

Changes to primary healthcare and the role of diagnostic consultancy

1
The past and the present

During the 18 years of our diagnostic consultancy work there have been significant changes in the overall context in which general practice is delivered. That pace of change looks set to continue. In sharing and developing what we have learned from visiting practices over that time, we have been very conscious of the need both to draw from the past and also to set our conclusions and lessons in the present and future context for primary care. This first chapter therefore starts with a brief discussion of that context.

Five principal changes can be summarised as follows:

1 **The changing nature of primary care**, as general practice and primary care have moved from being the point of entry and referral to the health system, to being major providers of care in their own right.

2 **The developing concept of partnership and team-working**, with much more emphasis on the non-medical contribution to healthcare delivery as chronic illness and preventative care are managed mainly in the community setting.

3 **Structural and political change**, as successive governments, the wider public and many in the health professions have started (although not finished) to shift the emphasis in healthcare from a professionally oriented to patient-oriented service.

4 **Increased accountability and the application of basic management method to clinical care, through the development of clinical governance**, embodying the principles of audit and external peer review against explicit professional standards.

5 **The development of the commissioning role** in respect of purchase of secondary care, with the management and organisational demands that entails.

Each of these changes is explored below.

The changing nature of primary care

The sort of care the public wants reflects the societal values and priorities current at any given time. In the 1970s and earlier, the emphasis was on secondary and tertiary care — the sexy, glossy and glamorous end of medicine, where miracles occurred. This is no longer so. The public now wants more accessible, 'user-friendly' care on its doorstep, as well as good secondary care. Primary care today is seen as the way of organising healthcare better through maintaining patients at home or in the community, where it is appropriate to do so, reflecting current social thinking and demand. General practice, the main provider of primary care, provides major services in early decisions about acute illness, in the care of the chronically sick and preventative medicine. In other words, there has been an important re-valuing of the rather 'messy and un-sexy part of the service' (Irvine and Irvine, 1996).

In the 1989 White Paper *Working for Patients* (DoH, 1989), and the *New Contract* which followed (DoH, 1990), determined (and, for many, misguided) attempts were made to strengthen accountability in general practice and to contain costs, especially of prescribing. At the same time, almost as an afterthought, general practice fundholding was introduced. This greatly extended the influence and power of those practices which took it up, through their ability to purchase secondary care. Arguably, however, the main impact of fundholding was on the practices themselves because of the new organisational and management demands it made. In particular, those at the leading edge used the enhanced practice management requirements to develop their capacity to quantify and monitor their care.

This trend has continued. Today, under a different government and a new NHS Act, the key elements of fundholding have been extended to all practices through the potential of the PCGs, LHGs and LHCs. In addition, there are completely new services such as NHS Direct, the walk-in clinics and nurse practitioner services.

For practices, this steady evolutionary trend points in one direction only. To be effective, indeed to survive, practices have got to get to grips with the key messages that flow from our observations over the years.

Partnership and the team

This change of role and position in the hierarchy of healthcare has put enormous demands on general practice and has forced changes in its way of working, particularly in relation to other members of the primary healthcare team. As Huxham (1993) said, 'Collaborative advantage will be achieved when something unusually creative is produced that no organisation could have produced on its own and when each organisation through collaboration is able to achieve its own objectives better than it could have done alone.'

As a consequence, multidisciplinary working in primary care has received a lot of attention in recent years. As Chapter 4 shows, it is still in transition but the lead role of medicine and the medical profession as the guardians of the nation's health, both population and individual, is now shared with others. The development of the wide range of skills and professions now involved in the delivery of healthcare has tested doctors in their management role and their attitudes to the development of wider partnerships, not just inside but outside the practice.

The development of group practice followed the 1966 Doctors' Charter as the first formalisation of the concept of partnership in healthcare — partnership between doctors. That soon extended with the attachment of district nurses and health visitors, and extended again with the arrival of practice nurses and the other health professionals with primary care responsibilities. Fundholding accelerated the rising position of managers in practice as significant members and, frequently, architects of the primary healthcare team. Full teamworking on practice development plans and inter-professional training has become commonplace. Case Study B in Chapter 8 shows how this can be done.

The concept of partnership and the statutory duty now imposed on healthcare trusts and authorities to seek and exercise partnership across boundaries are the latest in a series of changes in concepts of professional hierarchy (DoH, 2000). Doctors now have to be able to work effectively within wider organisations, such as PCGs, LHGs and LHCCs, and allied institutions, local councils and authorities, voluntary and charitable bodies, user and carer groups as well as the private sector. For instance, there are some areas where trusts responsible for mental health services and social services departments have found sufficient common ground and means of resolving the thorny problem of different funding streams to enable multidisciplinary and multi-agency teams to be formed. In some cases, for example, a community psychiatric nurse is accountable to a social worker (Northumberland Health Authority, 1999).

Structural and organisational reorientation

Alongside the changing nature of team-based care has been the change in emphasis from a professional to a patient-oriented service. This change in cultural orientation is not complete. That is why today we see some practices that regard the patient as the starting point for service while others still see the professional service as the primary driver. At a practical level this can result in important differences, for example in attitudes to patients, the way that complaints are handled or whether patient views are sought on practice services and performance, and so on.

In this changing climate, themes are developing around:

- more user-friendly care
- easier access largely through electronic technology developments
- wider range of healthcare delivered in or through the primary setting
- more emphasis on prevention
- increased multidisciplinary workforce
- greater use of professions other than doctors in independent settings
- greater integration with social care and social services
- more emphasis on cross-boundary working between primary and secondary care, especially in the management of chronic illness.

These structural and organisational changes in primary care mean that it is already – consciously or not – at the forefront of the government's modernisation agenda. The developments reflect, and will further reveal, issues and tensions that have been underlying the organisation and development of general practices since group practice became common. They can be summarised as:

- the capacity of primary care to deliver the expanded range of responsibilities and services

- the demand for efficient and provably efficacious services against the value of holistic and traditional family doctoring

- the conflict between uniformly and centrally driven high quality with the need for local flexibility and innovation

- the loss of the personal touch as more remote means of communications and support are offered

- the balance between vocational service and the modern values of private and family life.

These are difficult tensions to manage. They are exacerbated by the pressure created by other factors discussed below.

Most commentators see the government's White Paper *The New NHS* (DoH, 1997) as evolutionary rather than revolutionary. Many of the organisational and institutional changes we have described are intended to force changes in professional behaviour. Example 4 illustrates this.

Example 4

Basketball Surgery had been a first-wave fundholding practice. The six partners were enthusiastic supporters of the concepts involved in quality improvement and saw fundholding as a means of ensuring that patients obtained the best secondary care available through the placing of contracts by the practice. When fundholding was abandoned, the same partners saw PCGs, and the future PCTs, as an opportunity to further develop their potential to constrain and monitor the secondary care that the PCG, and through it the health authority, was commissioning for their patients. They saw the new developments as further enabling them in their advocacy and commissioning role.

Increased accountability and the development of clinical governance

Largely as a result of the development of teaching practices, the principles of external peer review against explicit professional standards have long been embodied in the culture of a substantial element of general practice. Teaching GPs were ahead of the government and the NHS in exploring the use of audit and quality assurance in the teaching practice setting.

The problem is that these basic principles of standard setting and monitoring were never extended to all general practices, either by the profession itself or by the NHS. This is now changing fast. The public demand for greater accountability, especially of professional performance, has brought performance assessment and quality assurance high on the professional and managerial agenda. At the time of writing clinical governance is being implemented and the GMC's revalidation plans, embracing audit and appraisal against explicit standards, are out for consultation. Chapter 6 explores this in the context of the underlying issues we have revealed through diagnostic consultancy.

Closing the gap between the extremes of variation in general practice needs a general change in both professional and institutional culture, with more emphasis on openness, a willingness to confront error and learn from it, and the adoption of the culture of quality improvement rather than blame. This substantial change implies an equally substantial programme of education, re-skilling and investment in the data and other systems which have to become part of the quality agenda. This is what clinical governance should be all about.

Quality is at the core and practices are going to have to keep pace. The statutory framework and the changed professional ethos that now inform quality mean that practices will be required to:

- submit themselves to annual appraisals based on *Duties of a Doctor: good medical practice* (GMC, 1995; RCGP, 1999)

- adhere to National Service Frameworks (NSFs) for the treatment of specified conditions, such as mental health and diabetes

- produce action plans in response to Commission for Health Improvement (CHI) visits

- have revalidation for GPs based on a folder of evidence of doctors' performance reviewed every five years, and for other professions within the practice team

- implement local health improvement plans (HImPs).

It is vital that GPs and their colleagues in primary care enter this new age with a clear knowledge and understanding of the strengths and weaknesses that their training and structures bring to patient care. Their experiences of the past in coming to grips with the problems around managing group practices and delivering care with restricted resources should strengthen their capacity to meet these challenges, given an awareness of the need to do so. The clinical governance agenda in the context of PCGs, LHGs and LHCs, and within practices themselves, give the opportunity to build on that foundation. Skills learnt in the past, and described in Chapters 3–6, will be essential.

A significant lever in the development of clinical governance and the changing role of primary care is the introduction of more explicit accountability. All professions are rightly held to account for the way they conduct their business. All professions are facing changes in the manner in which they are held to account (RCGP, 2000a).

There has been increasing recognition of the central roles that audit, performance review and self-appraisal play for a professional. The need to know what you are doing and be able to justify it to others. This is the 'black hole' or missing link, both inside and outside general practice, that will play the most important part in retaining and developing public confidence for

the future. However, some practitioners have little or no awareness of the existence, and therefore the importance, of these
performance issues.

This has underlined the fact that clinicians must account in
three ways – to themselves in their professional responsibilities, to the government as the paymaster, and to the public as
patients and carers. There has always been a tension in the way
these three perceive quality, producing what Øvretviet (1992)
described as 'the complex customer'. Some activities, such as
plastic surgery, may delight the patient but offend the Treasury;
the cure for the common cold may be a high priority for patients
but be low on the doctors' list; clinical professionals and patients
may see certainty of access to healthcare as a quality marker,
whereas the government may be more concerned with controlling waiting lists through the gatekeeper function of primary
care (Irvine and Irvine, 1996).

The accountability to colleagues and the collective profession
has had its outward visible signs for over the past 150 years in
the Royal Colleges and the General Medical Council. The
profession obtained and retained public trust and respect as its
capacity to identify and deal with disease, pain and suffering
increased. The reward was to be left alone. Government and
state accountability was almost non-existent. The setting up of
the NHS in 1948 changed that relationship between profession
and state, with the government being able to twitch the purse
strings much more actively, at least in the public sector.
However, until now, there has been little realistic accountability
to the state, and professional regulation or clinical autonomy
has been the bedrock of professional standards.

Increased public expectation has led to increasing involvement of patients and lay people in the management and accountability of the NHS. This is being matched by increasing public
involvement in professional regulation so that now it is professionally led regulation rather than professional self-regulation
(RCGP, 2000a). The medical profession is seeking to meet the
legitimate demands of the patients and society as a whole, while

not giving up the crucial freedoms that enable doctors to advocate freely for their patients, particularly where de facto clinical rationing is in operation.

But public trust is demonstrably the key to political arrangements between medicine, society and the state (Salter, 1999), and the exposure of the major clinical failures – Bristol, Kent and Canterbury, Ledward, Shipman and Neale – of the past few years have put the public's trust in that bedrock at risk.

There have been other developments that have undermined that public trust and/or changed the nature of the one-to-one relationship of doctor and patient in the privacy of the consulting room that has been the foundation of professional accountability.

These include:

- a general decline in the authority and legitimacy of all professions in society

- the increased accessibility of medical knowledge, particularly through electronic technology and the Internet

- increased complaints and lobbies

- the increased dependence of medicine on skills and technologies outside its control and knowledge base, such as in the field of genetics

- the rise of the salaried GP and consequent loss of continuity of family care

- the development of the 'professional' locum

- the rise of complementary medicine.

The history of the past 18 years of our experience with general practice gives valuable lessons for the future. These are dealt with in Chapter 6 and the practical implications of it are illustrated in Case Study C in Chapter 9.

The development of the commissioning role and increased management demands

Fundholding and now groups, trusts and boards have led to an enhanced role in the commissioning of secondary services. This in itself has exacerbated the already significant problem most GPs have had with the concepts and activities involved in the effective management of an organisation and its people. The RCGP has set out what this means in terms of good general practice (RCGP, 1999). The key support for the delivery of this remains what it has always been – the medical profession's capacity to handle the management of the primary care organisation, and in particular people working within it. Of overriding significance is the ability to develop good relationships and a collective will to self-manage (GMC, 1995).

The development of awareness of this vital aspect of the GP's role has been slow and painful. Awareness has usually come from the individual practice as a result of a crisis of resource, morale or external pressure, combined with tightened employment legislation, particularly from Brussels. It is still a struggle for medical education to include a significant element that increases the sensitivity of students to other professionals and colleagues, or help them to apply the largely common sense that makes up good management at the practice level. Skill levels and awareness have mostly improved because of the modelling often provided by practice managers. The management expertise of these members of the primary healthcare team was increased dramatically by fundholding, although perversely the management skills needed to manage these high-level managers has itself put pressure on general practice.

General practice services are traditionally demand-led and therefore they are not well-placed in general to take a strategic view and take on a population-based approach to health promotion and development. An evaluation of total purchasing pilots for instance showed that little use was made of health needs assessment or evidence of effectiveness to inform purchasing decisions (Arora *et al.*, 2000). But there have been many GPs looking for ways of taking their practice forward, those whom Bosanquet calls 'innovators' (Bosanquet and Leese, 1989). They have been receptive to outside expertise and to subject it to an independent expert appraisal and assess its fitness for its purpose. Such an experience leads to an awareness of the need for change and how to achieve it for the benefit of the practice and its patient. The examples in Chapters 3–6 illustrate this experience.

The dominance of GPs within most PCGs, LHGs and LHCs makes them liable for their success or failure, and will determine the sort of role they are able to play in the very different PCTs as they are formed in England. The art will be to manage primary care in a way that reduces practice variation and enhances quality openly and efficiently, while leaving the independent contractor status of the GP untouched. Delivery of the primary care reforms envisaged needs a clearly articulated objective, shrewd management and careful performance assessment (Bloor *et al.*, 1999). Above all, it needs skills in managing ways of working together effectively for an increasingly wide range of contributors to healthcare. In these circumstances, the changes in partnership and teamworking in general practice have been significant to date, and look set fair to continue to be so.

Conclusion

The current changes and challenges in the health scene described here do not detract from the lessons to be learnt from the past, but rather enhance them. The sort of diagnostic lessons arising from practice visits of the kind undertaken by the authors are of particular relevance to the change agenda of tomorrow.

These challenges resonate throughout this book as the issues found through diagnostic analysis of individual practice are described and the ways of handling them discussed.

2
What is diagnostic consultancy?

Diagnostic consultancy is similar to the process of a clinical consultation. It attempts to establish the true underlying problems that beset a practice in the same way the clinician looks for the underlying causes of presenting illness in the consulting room. It is, of course, concerned primarily with organisational matters, individual and group attitudes and behaviour. But these are inextricably tied in with the delivery of clinical care.

Diagnostic consultancy reveals the strengths and weaknesses of organisations by helping their members see how the organisation works, its people and their relationships, and the obstacles to future development. It provides a capacity to translate these observations into coherent patterns and present them in a way most likely to bring about understanding within the organisation. In particular, it highlights how little people really know about each other's motivations. It helps the participants to confront difficult situations in a positive way and therefore achieve change without being so confrontational as to be self-defeating.

Diagnostic consultancy is a prime example of the adage 'The outsider sees more of the game'. It usually starts from a request to help solve a presenting problem. A practice identifies a need or concern which they feel can best be explored by using an external source. The sort of problems put forward in this way are described more fully in Chapter 3. These concerns may come from all the partners working together on their future plans, from one or two who are frustrated or thwarted by others, from the practice manager or any combination of the three. More recently, it has come from a health authority worried about the apparent non-performance of a practice.

The diagnostic process

The following is a brief résumé of the processes involved in a diagnostic consultancy visit. Appendix A gives a detailed account and Case Studies A and C in Chapters 7 and 9 describe two such visits.

The process is in five parts:

1   The consultancy starts with a pre-visit discussion between the commissioner(s) of the visit and the consultants to clarify the purpose of the review and to identify the key players from the commissioners' point of view.

2   The diagnostic visit is arranged and the timetable for interviews is finalised.

3   Interviews with partners and staff to obtain and test views are the central part of the visit. Not only are they the principal means of gathering information about the dynamics of the practice, but they also present developmental opportunities through discussion.

4   Early initial conclusions and possible options for the way forward are offered in verbal feedback at the end of the visit.

5   A subsequent full written report sets out in tangible form the findings of the visit, as well as the more mature reflections of the consultants as to the possible ways forward.

Often the ways forward suggested by the diagnostic process require additional external support, such as longer-term follow-up after a period.

The outcomes

The benefits of such visits can take years to be felt fully, but there are four principal outcomes to highlight here.

1 Identifying the real, as distinct from the presenting, issues in practices

When things go wrong most practices forget their strengths. They may seize on a range of sometimes fairly superficial manifestations to explain defined and undefined feelings of disharmony and dissatisfaction. Alternatively, they may point to immediate apparent reasons for specific problems, such as high staff turnover, poor morale, loss of income, heavy workload. Case Studies A, C and D in Chapters 7, 9 and 10 give some examples of the issues presented over the years. The issues are discussed here under six headings:

- partners
- policies
- the practice manager
- management expertise
- staff
- the structures and environment.

Partners

One of the most common problems that practices identify as the root of their ills is lack of time. This is often related to a heavy workload and/or over-demanding patients. Often the two things go together with a resulting aggressive response to patient demand. Partners may complain about colleagues not starting on time or keeping to time. This, in turn, can be linked to a belief that the appointment system needs review and the way of handling extras needs to be changed. This is often related to a perceived disparity of workload between partners, for instance with a new partner who cannot cope with the retiring partner's workload. The use of half and whole days off per week and other external activities can mean a loss of doctor time for appointments and put more pressure on appointment times.

Some practices recognise themselves that their inability to progress as a practice is often due to dysfunctional partnership, which may be linked to a recognised vacuum in leadership within the partner group. This can often be coupled with, at one extreme, anxiety about the autocracy of senior partners or, at the other, about anarchy because no one can decide who should take the lead when necessary. This indecisiveness or apparent extreme difference of view may be identified as the cause of an inability to agree priorities for the practice and devise future strategies for practice.

This lack of a common view can be reflected in a paralysis over the appointment of new partners. The need to replace a practice manager can reveal a lack of common view among partners about the sort of replacement needed, or a lack of confidence in the practice's selection process.

Policies

Practices frequently cite too much change, both external and internal, as a real problem, resulting in an inability to keep changing practice policies to manage the change effectively. Latterly, they have also identified a lack of representation on PCGs, LHGs or LHCCs as a reason for current or future difficulty.

The practice manager

One of the most common reasons put forward by practices for their perceived ills is the inadequacy of the practice's management. Partners usually see this as reflecting not on the partnership, but on the practice manager. Often, where a manager has been promoted from the staff, it can be perceived that the practice has developed faster than the practice manager or beyond his/her competence. This may be related in some instances to partners' concerns about increasing costs of staff and the resultant impact on their drawings.

Poor systems, often around the issues of time management and appointments systems, are frequently laid at the door of the practice manager. Similarly, complaints and concerns about the increased paperwork generated internally or externally are often blamed on management.

Some practices see the practice manager as integral to the partnership and a major source of management support and advice, but this can slide into concerns that the manager has become over-mighty. This is particularly the case where new partners, who were not party to the original appointment, want change and see the practice manager as blocking their efforts.

Management expertise

Rarely do partners identify their own limitations as a problem — certainly not in terms of management skills. Their lack of organisational experience becomes obvious when, for instance, a vacancy for a practice manager occurs. The partners may find that they are unable to agree on the job description or the nature of the role that they want to delegate to the new practice manager.

Staff

A practice can see poor morale of staff as a worrying sign of poor organisational health in the practice. Equally, poor performance by non-clinical staff can be used as a reason for poor performance of the practice generally.

The structures and environment

Poor premises as such are not often used as a presenting issue, though occasionally the existing branch surgeries are perceived as having a deleterious effect.

Example 5 further illustrates the benefit of identifying the real issues.

Example 5

The doctors in a five-partner practice in a semi-urban area of England were worried by the number of complaints they were receiving from patients about both long waiting times for appointments and unhelpful and incompetent receptionists. The partners worked in quite different ways, did not have common values or ways of working and demanded that each individual style be catered for. They saw the problems in terms of the competency of the practice manager. Although she was very experienced, she was rather unassertive. The partners sought external advice on how to remove her to bring in someone who could 'sort things out'.

The practice manager was clear that the real problems were with the availability of doctor time, and with the lack of money invested in receptionists' training and pay. However, she was not comfortable confronting the partners with this. The external review supported her view and the recommendation was that the partners look to resolve their differences in style and priorities first *and then* in the light of that, assess the reasons for the patients' complaints.

---

2   Moving the practice forward

Diagnostic consultancy is also good at finding ways of helping a practice move forward when the team feels blocked. Example 6 shows one case.

Example 6

Jean and Robert Taylor has founded Small Town Surgery 20 years ago. Robert was still the full-time senior partner and Jean was a part-time partner. They owned the premises and leased it to the partnership. There were now three other partners who felt increasingly stifled and constrained by the autocratic role played by Robert and the built-in veto he and Jean exercised on any ideas to change and develop. In particular, the premises were now far too small for the development of full teamworking, particularly in relation to expanding nursing services, plus the demands of health and safety legislation for the conditions in which staff worked.

One partner knew a health and safety expert and got her to review the practice's compliance. Her worrying report forced the partners to agree to a full external diagnostic review to identify all the areas where the partnership was at risk in terms of litigation, and where it was falling behind in terms of services, likely demands from the PCG and clinical governance. The diagnostic review revealed the full extent of the partners' frustrations and enabled a full disclosure and discussion of the issues holding the practice back.

3 Creating an effective team

A consultancy process such as the one described can also help a practice to gain clarity about the problems it faces, and how to address them, as Example 7 shows.

Example 7

Shawcross Medical Centre was a three-partner practice in the middle of a small town on the outskirts of an industrial area of Scotland. The partners and practice manager all got on very well, socially and professionally. They were very keen not to upset the good relationships and good atmosphere in the practice. However, they also knew that they were not good at handling poor or less-than-optimum performance at any level – doctor, manager, nurse or receptionist. They were aware of real problems in this area and felt unable to solve their dilemma. They sought external help.

The external consultant used the interviews she held to bring into the open, in a safe environment, the irritations and frustrations felt by all but which none wanted to express. The one-to-one interviews helped them individually to recognise that confronting issues did not have to be aggressive or damaging, but could be constructive and helpful. An 'away day' for the practice was held, facilitated by the consultant, at which these views and concerns were debated openly. The protected environment meant that they felt able to share ideas and thoughts, and disagree with each other, without the atmosphere degenerating into the sort of unpleasantness they had all feared, or their relationships being fundamentally harmed.

4 Revealing practice strengths

The benefits of diagnostic consultancy include creating a change of culture and the release of energy and ideas in a practice. In particular, the process can help to identify and underline the strengths of a practice which can often be forgotten.

There is a tendency when practices are reviewing their problems, and particularly when asked by external reviewers to assess the practice's strengths and weaknesses, to overstate the issues of concern. They often present a picture of all being 'rotten in the state of Denmark'. It is important for the consultant to help the partners set what can appear to be overwhelming weaknesses in perspective. This is done by identifying the clear strengths and giving back confidence to all those working within the organisation. The starting point for all stages of the review is, therefore, to remind the practice of the foundation on which it is building. In this way, the subsequent catalogue of areas of concern or for development can be measured appropriately. This is not just a cynical 'stroking' exercise to legitimise the coming revelations, but part of helping the members of the practice learn to look honestly at the business and the people working in it.

The first obvious strength of any practice in this position is the fact that external consultants are there at all reviewing its activities, either clinical or non clinical. This shows considerable courage and insight. It also invariably reflects other areas of achievement which can be highlighted prior to analysing the presenting and underlying issues that may be holding the organisation back or making it demoralised and unhappy.

These other sources of pride and satisfaction can include the stability and longevity of the partnership, and the common values and philosophy held. Regular meetings, regular audits and a systematic approach to identifying areas for improvements may be part of these strengths. The practice manager may be a strength both through their role in establishing and maintaining good relationships with staff and partners, and also their contribution to the ideas and development of the practice. The partners may have delegated management responsibilities effectively both within the partnership and to the practice manager and the staff team. Regular appraisal may be integral to the practice's management systems, and employment practices may be frequently reviewed and updated.

Staff can be a strength by being long-serving and well-motivated. They may be willing to work flexible hours and work as a team. The premises may be well-maintained with good facilities and equipment. Appendix B gives a more comprehensive list of possible practice strengths identified over the years.

In all the practices we have visited over the past 18 years, those working in the practice have presented firm ideas as to the problem or problems as they see them. As the following chapters make clear, invariably the practice visit has revealed quite different underlying issues.

Part 2
Underlying issues

Introduction

As happens in a clinical consultation, there are often more fundamental causes for problems in practice than the immediate presenting symptoms. Many of them relate to attitude and culture within the practice and their influence on patient care.

> ## Example 8
>
> The Melton Practice took part in a research programme establishing the views of patients about a range of issues relating to patient services. The patient questionnaires showed that the most important aspects of care from the patient point of view were in key areas of access and timekeeping, and also a consistency of approach between partners and nurses, an appearance of efficiency, a friendly atmosphere and a caring, professional attitude throughout the practice. In all these areas, Melton Practice came out badly, although it was generally accepted that the clinical care was good. The practice was astonished as its own analysis of its problems was about workload, staff turnover and keeping up with clinical developments.

Example 8 reflects the main underlying issues that have been identified through diagnostic consultancy, and which are as true and relevant today as they were 18 years ago. They are discussed under four main headings:

1   divergent and unspoken philosophies and values (Chapter 3)

2   limited management awareness and skill (Chapter 4)

3   difficulties in working across boundaries, within and outside practice (Chapter 5)

4   acceptance and delivery of accountability to self and others (Chapter 6).

The following chapters elaborate each and include some of the ways forward that have been found to be effective. The chapters cross-refer to the case studies in Part 3, which illustrate the themes further.

3
Common philosophy and values

Introduction

The most significant change that has occurred in the way medicine is delivered in primary care over the past 18 years is the transformation from seeing the service and its practitioners as the centre of the practice activities to putting the needs of patients first. The rate of this change varies across practices and doctors. It is not surprising therefore that the most common underlying problem that we have identified in that time often revolves around whether or not there are common values and philosophies in the practice. These values and philosophies span a range of often unspoken and unarticulated taboo areas, such as the place of money in the practice's value system, attitudes to patients or attitudes to clinically questionable practice. Such unspoken, but often fundamentally divergent, values can be underlined and reinforced by inadequate communication between partners, and by poor communications strategies. These may include no regular, structured and protected meetings because of pressure of work, such as illustrated in Case Study C in Chapter 9.

The fact that these tensions may remain unspoken and not confronted can be the result of people not wanting to rock the boat or open up likely areas of discomfort. This may be because of an unspoken lack of confidence in the partnership. This can be coupled with an unwillingness to handle the emotional discomfort or even turmoil that confronting problems can bring.

As a result, partners may avoid handling basic issues where their individual values and beliefs appear to diverge. A common consequence of such collusive relationships can be that the partnership does not confront performance matters effectively, either in each other or in staff.

Such collusion can also be the result of not planning ahead, and sometimes be a symptom of it. In order to decide on future areas of development and priority, a practice needs to agree on what are its current priorities. Rather than face the differences that might emerge or may be revealed through this process, practices often just avoid the planning at all, thus depriving themselves doubly. The effect of this is to make it difficult for practice members to scan the horizon for likely changes in healthcare, which will affect them. This paralysis in planning can lead to the reactive practice, which is unhappy because it cannot influence its own destiny. Equally, such practices are not good at testing themselves against other practices, not least to bring in new developments and ideas.

A common direction

Being clear about personal values and the work ethics of colleagues is not just a modern management fad. It is fundamental to anticipating problems before they arise, spotting the controversial issues and planning ways of dealing with them, and providing a framework within which all participants can work and direct their energies. Yet in our experience it is still unusual even in the best practices today. Case Studies C and D both demonstrate these problems.

One way of checking whether all agree on values and philosophies is by putting each partner's and, where appropriate, each practice member's personal motivations and goals on the table, and talking through the differences and similarities revealed. The sorts of question to be asked are summarised in Box 3.1 together with the most common answers.

Box 3.1: Personal motivations and goals

1 Why are you in this organisation?
- I want to serve the community.
- I want to improve the health of patients.
- It fits my personality type.
- It helps me be independent.
- It gives me the opportunity to follow my particular interests, e.g. research.
- It gives me status (in the family, in the community).
- It gives me an easy life.
- I make a good living.

2 How would you rank the following in your life?
- Job.
- Time.
- Money.
- Health
- Family.
- Other interests.

3 How would you rank the following as priorities in your work?
- Service to patients.
- Your professional development.
- Your income.
- Your non-work time.

Without this base line of information, complete misunderstandings and seriously wrong assumptions affecting the whole future of the practice can result, as demonstrated in Example 9.

Example 9

A group of five partners in an inner-city practice had a good day-to-day working relationship. They met little outside the practice, and only for business meetings inside. But they felt they knew each other's motivations and personal agendas well enough to take them on trust. The partnership talked at length about the external roles of three of them, Jim as chair of the PCG, Clare as secretary of the local medical committee (LMC) and John as a GP tutor and trainer. Paula, a fourth partner, now asked the partners if she could have a sabbatical to complete her doctorate. The fifth partner, George, had no outside interests, but had a heavy list, worked very hard, never refused to see extras and always agreed to stand in for last-minute problems with surgeries. Jim, Clare and John all agreed that Paula could take the three months off, and turned to George, assuming he would agree to carry the larger part of the workload. He always had, and anyway they believed he was devoted to his patients and to being a family doctor.

To their astonishment, not only did he say no, but announced that, as he was reaching 50 the following year, he was giving notice of his intention to retire and buy a yacht to take chartered trips to the Mediterranean. The partners had no knowledge of his interest in sailing, and certainly not of his plans to retire early. They asked him if he would miss the patients. He further astonished them by saying that he was indifferent to the patients. He was bored by general practice and saw it merely as a job to do as well as he could until he had sufficient money to do what really turned him on.

As a result of years of making huge assumptions about each other and never testing values and philosophies, the partnership found itself in considerable difficulties. Paula was able to take time out, but Jim had to resign as chair of the PCG and Clare had to cut back her role as secretary of the LMC. However, one of the greatest difficulties they faced individually and as a group was that George's revelations undermined their opinion of themselves as thoughtful, caring and perceptive people.

The second step is to get everyone to declare their aims and perceptions of the direction in which they want the organisation to go in the next few years. They can do this by offering their answers to the questions set out in Box 3.2.

Box 3.2: Organisational aims and direction

1 What should be the priorities for the organisation for the next three years?
2 What will be the measures of success for achieving these priorities?
3 What are the main obstacles to achieving these aims?

The agreement of all parties to a statement of common aim and direction is the outward visible sign of an organisation handling the task of establishing an articulated and agreed common philosophy and value base. Developing an agreed or common direction is not done by magic. It takes time, and can be tough and hard as the extended example of Case Study D in Chapter 10 demonstrates. The mistake some organisations make is to believe that it must be innovative; what is crucial is not originality but how well it serves the interests of the constituents, the level of commitment all owners feel for it, and how closely it reflects and complements their personal goals. The value lies in the process gone through to achieve it, its publication, and the framework it provides for the whole organisation to work within and towards.

In moving forward, practices have found it helpful to test themselves against the following questions:

- do we all know and empathise with each other's values?

- do we make the opportunities to discuss them and identify differences?

- do we all agree that it is worthwhile reviewing regularly the common philosophy underlying the practice culture to make sure the consensus still holds?

- do we all agree on the general direction in which the organisation should develop?

Managing and confronting known differences and past baggage

Openness is essential to establishing where everyone is coming from and going to, and in handling the articulation of any differences revealed. Yet in our experience, real openness is exceptional. A group of people working together can be rife with politics, unspoken feelings, fears and tensions. One of the reasons why the answers to some of the questions posed on page 39 may be negative, is a lack of confidence in many groups to handle the potential conflict or disagreement that may be revealed. It takes a considerable effort to reveal hidden agendas and to express feelings, to trust one's colleagues and to speak one's mind.

The pace of change in primary care has increased, together with the range of areas of conflict and disagreement, and both will undoubtedly continue to do so. Issues such as unacceptable behaviour generated by outmoded beliefs in gender and race, and differences or fundamental conflicts of values and goals, need to be aired positively at all levels. This may be between partners in a practice, doctors working together in a local health group, nurses working in a community team or managers delivering the organisational framework for a PCG. So this question of openness about values and attitudes has got to be grasped.

Example 10 illustrates a common area of conflict – that of tensions between the practice as a business and the practice as a caring 'social' service. This particular example derives from the era of fundholding, but in our experience the issue of fundholding was frequently the catalyst for revealing much more deep-seated tensions.

Example 10

Three of the six partners in the Shepherd Surgery were positive about the benefits to patients to be derived from fundholding. Another felt that it was primarily a test of GPs' abilities to operate as business managers. The other two partners had fundamental philosophical objections to being involved in the commissioning of what they saw as two-tier care. They saw the handing over of detailed activity information to government as subversive and an intrusion on clinical and personal freedoms. The discussions about the proposal to seek fundholding status were not, however, open and constructive but consisted of many three-way discussions among the partners who were keen and blank vetoes by the two who did not want to go forward in this way.

As a result, the practice did not develop fundholding but the relations between the partners deteriorated so badly that they were unable to discuss anything beyond holiday rotas. Patient care began to suffer, staff morale plummeted and the practice income began to fall. Eventually one partner retired, and the youngest partner and practice manager both resigned because of the atmosphere of unresolved and unacknowledged conflict. The remaining partners called in external consultants to help them talk through what was happening, and to help them dispose of the past baggage they were all carrying.

To handle the sort of disharmony in Example 10 individuals/the group need to be helped to recognise that a constructive outcome is fundamental. There is a need therefore to recognise that there is a difference between the opposing views themselves and the hostile feelings that can result. Criticism and arguments need to be about the ideas or behaviour, what people believe and do, not about personality or what they are.

It is important to understand and recognise the difference between destructive conflict, as illustrated in Example 10, and the sort of positive tension that can abound for instance when choosing a new partner or testing the value of a new piece of equipment. In the latter cases, creative tension can be vital to generating ideas, enhancing understanding and maintaining the momentum to move the organisation forward.

The best way of handling disruptive conflict or hindering behaviour is before hostilities break out. The suggested ways forward for a group are:

- to meet regularly

- to consult all interested parties before making decisions that affect them

- to avoid criticising each other in front of others

- to praise and support publicly

- to confront openly and non-aggressively issues that have to be dealt with, however unpleasant.

Case Study D in Chapter 10 describes one way of helping a practice to face up to difficult issues in a protected environment.

If all these ploys fail, or if the issue is about long-standing behaviour such as bullying by a partner of staff, then conflict must be faced. Example 11 shows how.

Example II

In a four-doctor partnership, the chair, Stewart, was a bully and a tyrant. He was thoroughly unpleasant to the staff — belittling them in front of patients, shouting down the telephone at them when interrupted in surgery and abusing them roundly if they asked him to see extra patients. In between these moments of being offensive, he was charm personified! Most of the staff were long-serving and long-suffering. They believed that in spite of his rude and arrogant behaviour he was a good doctor, kind to his patients, and the only partner with drive and initiative.

A new practice manager was appointed and was horrified at this workplace harassment of both staff and younger partners, two of whom were female job-sharers. At a partners' meeting she tried to raise the issue by referring to the importance of privacy within the reception area for patients, but also for the staff and doctors. Although she had spoken to all the partners about the chair's behaviour beforehand, when the issue arose, none of them attempted to support her or were as honest as they had been on a one-to-one basis. On the contrary, it was made clear to her that she was overstepping the mark by raising it.

The issue was not debated fully, partly out of fear of Stewart's response but also because most felt that Stewart had given years of service to the practice and should be indulged. The practice manager felt bruised and let down, although she remained clear that she had been right to raise it. As they had not pursued the matter in what she felt would have been a constructive way, she felt she had to put her cards on the table more forcibly. She told the partners that they needed to establish a clear policy around the treatment of practice members. Above all, such a policy should reflect the need to treat all members of the team with respect, to deal with complaints in private initially and not to use status or gender to exercise power. If they did not, then she believed the practice was exposed to the avoidable risk of legal action for workplace harassment.

As this stark reality dawned on them, the partners realised the situation was serious. Stewart denied any inappropriate behaviour on his part. However, the partners decided to draw a practice policy for good relations and an anti-harassment agreement to which they would all have to subscribe. They avoided blaming Stewart but made it clear that any person in the practice transgressing the new policy would be subject to disciplinary action and, if a partner, to exclusion from the partnership.

Case Studies C and D in Chapters 9 and 10 demonstrate that failure to confront when necessary is one of the commonest causes of problems in general practice. This could get worse in PCGs as the opportunities to avoid the issue and conceal such issues in the mass will be greater.

Avoiding conflict therefore includes denying it exists, side-stepping it or – the most common response – procrastination. There are two other principal reactions. The first is to try to defuse conflict and the second is to confront it head on. Defusing may involve avoiding the major points of contention and dealing only with the minor ones. For instance, if a partner is being rude and insulting to staff when they ask for help in dealing with extras, other partners may try to defuse the issue by changing the surgery rotas rather than dealing with the attitudinal change that is needed. This may be effective in the short term and may smooth things over, but only delay the final confrontation, as Example 11 showed.

Confronting in a constructive way is the only effective response. There are several ways of doing this without war breaking out. They can be divided into short- and long-term strategies.

Short-term strategies

Strategies that can be used for immediate, but essentially short-term, results include persuading people to change a specific habit, such as smoking, or negotiating a short-term compromise between two warring factions. Often this has a 'patching' effect only, as Example 12 shows.

Example 12

A health visitor persisted in smoking in the offices of the PCG, despite the building and the site having been recently designated a non-smoking zone. One of the staff made a formal complaint to the chair of the PCG and requested that urgent action be taken. The chair offered to put up more no-smoking notices and to see the health visitor to persuade her to stop.

The member of staff recognised that it was a difficult situation and accepted these interim ideas, as long as she was confident that 'management' would think out longer-term and more permanent solutions. She believed that it should be a disciplinary offence to smoke in a non-smoking area. In the end it was agreed, albeit reluctantly, that smokers would be allowed to smoke in the car park of the PCG offices.

Clearly in this case a win–win solution was only possible with compromise on all sides. A 'win–win' is always the desirable result, so that both sides can feel good. Resolving a conflict where both sides or one side feel put down, diminished, penalised, demoralised or having sustained some kind of loss is only storing up trouble for the future. The aim must be to arrive at a situation where the needs of both sides are met, where the organisation is viewed by its members in a favourable light and where confidence is gained in the ability of the organisation to resolve future conflicts quickly.

Long-term strategies

These are generally best as they are most likely to achieve the desired 'win–win' state. Example 13 is an example of where taking the longer view gives a chance to achieve this.

Example 13

In a large urban practice the practice manager, Jane, had been in post for 23 years, working with the original partner as general factotum. As the practice grew so Jane grew with it, and took the title 'practice manager' very early in this development. She was a patient of the practice. She was competent and knew the patients very well. She was not very skilled in handling staff and was averse to change of any kind, which she saw as merely resulting in more work.

As new partners arrived, Jane's base became less secure and she became more obstructive and negative. The senior partner, who was her registered doctor, tried to defend her on all occasions and several of the longer-serving staff, including the senior practice nurse, were supportive of her. They felt she had given faithful service to the practice, and in any case her knowledge of the practice area and the individual patients was invaluable to the health of the practice.

The newer partners frequently complained about her among themselves. They felt frustrated and resentful. Yet when they arrived at breaking point, they were held back because they dwelt immediately on the problem of how to remove her safely. The patients would be up in arms, the other staff would be incensed and some of the older ones might leave, she herself would make a fuss and the senior partner would support her. They would also lose a lot of vital information that no one else had. They wondered how they would replace her and especially how they would afford a new breed of practice manager – she had been, after all, very cheap.

Eventually they sought external advice. The consultant pointed out to them that they needed to work through what sort of practice they wanted and then describe the kind of management such a practice would need. Only then could they decide how much of that management they wanted to do themselves and how much they wished to delegate. From

> that would come a clear idea of the sort of skills needed and whether they had such skills in their current practice manager. If not, they had then to decide with her whether she could acquire them through training or redesigning her job, or whether there was such a new element in the post it was creating a redundancy situation. They recognised that uncomfortable though this process might be, it should meet most people's needs and was essential if the practice was to thrive and survive.

A number of techniques can be employed to achieve a 'win–win' situation:

- get people to put aside their individual needs for the greater good of the organisation
- get both sides to surrender something tangible and visible
- negotiate a situation where both parties gain something while neither gives up anything vital.

Leadership and negotiation are the tools and Box 3.3 sets out the essentials of a framework for successful negotiation.

Box 3.3: A framework for negotiation

- Achieve solutions from which both sides can benefit.
- Develop a belief that the other person in the conflict is a potential partner, not an adversary.
- Develop a climate in which both parties realise that their objectives can be obtained more by working together than working separately.
- Facilitate the process of securing mutual advantage for both parties.

In summary, therefore, handling conflict well is about being able to answer positively the following questions:

- do we know our differences?
- do we trust each other?

- who or what does each of us fear in confronting known differences or behaviours in others?

- do we have a clear and accurate understanding of each other?

Aggression and the exercise of power

In order to arrive at common philosophies and values, or to resolve differences, it is important to be able to distinguish between being assertive and being aggressive. For women in particular this can be a significant problem, as assertiveness can be labelled aggressiveness in order to de-feminise an assertive woman. Maintaining a firm line, particularly with a senior and older male colleague, can require considerable strength of purpose and coolness of temperament for a female partner or practice manager. Similarly, new partners, non-medical staff and nurses can feel inhibited from handling conflict in an assertive way, and that uncertainty can in itself lead to an appearance of aggression.

Box 3.4 sets out some tips for all those involved in such situations.

Box 3.4: Key skills of assertiveness

- Be clear what the problem is that you are trying to deal with and what changes you are trying to negotiate.
- State clearly and directly if and when you disagree, giving specific examples of and evidence for your views.
- Use legitimate criticism to help the other person, not to put them down.
- Describe behaviour, do not label the person.
- Recognise other people's points of view.
- Distinguish between fact and opinion.
- Give helpful feedback, summarising any agreements that have been reached.
- Recognise and believe in your right to disagree with someone.

However, besides handling such situations well, it is helpful to understand where the roots of aggression may lie. For many people, particularly where they are in any kind of subordinate role, fear is at the root avoiding confrontation with others. Much of this fear is rooted in the way power is exercised in any organisation. The concepts of power are explained fully elsewhere (Irvine and Irvine, 1996), but it is important to restate the key elements.

There are four main sources of power in an organisation. The first is that which comes from the position or status attaching to a title or function. For instance, any job title including the word 'senior' or 'head' carries with it an implication of greater power than those without. Care should be taken, therefore, in so designating, as Examples 14 and 15 show.

Example 14

In a semi-urban practice of six partners, the longest-serving partner, Peter, was very unwilling to be the chair of the partnership. He did not want to take on the responsibility and did not feel skilled in any of the tasks his partners expected him to take on as a result of the title.

As a result he took refuge in solitude, making decisions without consulting, telling rather than asking, setting agendas without consent and staying out of the staff common room where all the practice gathered. When challenged, he said that the partners had asked him to take the role of chair of the partnership and he felt that that meant he had a lot of difficult decisions to make. Too close a relationship with staff and colleagues would make those decisions all the harder. He felt he had to withdraw to stay neutral and be a detached leader. He swung from remoteness and indecision to authoritarianism and over-firm commitments on behalf of the whole partnership. He began to enjoy the power that the position and title gave him. The other partners felt powerless to remove the power from him.

Example 15

Judith was a long-service receptionist in the Shade Surgery. She was within three years of retirement and the partners wanted to give her additional remuneration to bump up her pension. They hit on the idea of calling her senior receptionist and gave her an extra 50p an hour. They did not change her job description or her duties. Two things happened. The other receptionists were up in arms as they felt it was unfair to effectively create a new post and not have open competition for it, particularly as it carried more money. But second, Judith took the word 'senior' seriously. She started to dictate to the others about the rota, appraisals and practice processes. In turn, because she had the title, the partners tended to dump all the difficulties on her to sort out. The partners regretted giving the trappings of power to Judith without thinking it through carefully enough. The practice had an uncomfortable three years and high turnover of staff until she retired.

The situations set out in the above examples are hopefully becoming rarer nowadays, as in most organisations the position or status of a person frequently does not give them absolute power to command others. This probably only still exists in the uniformed services. It does, however, allow the office-holder to call meetings, to apply processes and procedures as agreed by everybody, and to stop things happening. In dealing with confrontation, therefore, it is often helpful to have a person designated as 'executive manager' or 'grievance/complaints manager'. Often in practice this is the practice manager, who can then, by virtue of office, confront others assertively and confidently.

The second area in which power is exercised is where the individual or individuals hold the purse strings (as where a partner owns the premises from which the practice works) or control resources in some way. That means the person will be able to facilitate or prevent something from happening by the provision or withholding of resources. The partners can give or withhold pay increases, provide equipment, and hire and fire. Clearly, however, resource power is a negotiable commodity, because of the need for collaboration and support throughout the team.

The third way in which power is exercised is through specialised expertise and knowledge. This is perhaps the most common in practices in which there are many in the team with specific and arcane areas of technical and jargon-riddled specialism, from the doctors and nurses, through to computer operators and managers, and beyond the practice to bank managers and accountants. Doctors, in spite of erosions of their positions and status in recent years, still retain special expertise and, therefore, power in healthcare. But besides nurses and other therapists gaining power in specific areas of clinical activity, managers too are gaining in expert power. This becomes increasingly obvious as PCGs develop and demand high levels of managerial expertise.

Lastly, there is the increasingly important element of power, known as personal power. This is what a person brings to the task in hand. It includes things such as charisma, manner, style and presence — all those intangibles that create a sense of significant attributes, which are difficult to challenge. Strong leaders can exercise this very effectively, even where there are strong downsides to his or her skill base. Example 16 illustrates this.

Example 16

John was elected chair of the Downshire LHG. He was a GP of 20 years' standing, a national figure in the development of multidisciplinary working in practice and coming from a practice with a high reputation for good clinical care. He had written extensively on general practice, had been awarded an MBE and was, in addition, a big man physically with a strong voice and considerable presence.

He was, however, a hopeless manager of people. His practice had a high turnover of staff because he was an unconscious bully. His voice startled and frightened receptionists and junior partners alike. He was very clear of his own priorities and those of the practice, and was unaware of anyone else's doubts.

In the practice, his colleagues had learned to collude with this behaviour and keep the peace. In the LHG, however, his personal power position was not recognised so much. His fellow board members and the chief executive were all strong personalities with clear ideas, which they wanted to share and discuss. His rather autocratic and dictatorial manner, albeit not intended to offend, did not sit happily with the consensus politics and partnership approach engendered by his LHG colleagues. He was confronted firmly and assertively by the vice chair and the chief executive, who clearly stated the areas of concern, the strengths and the positive points about his chairmanship, but also the ways in which he had to change. He had never been confronted in this way before, and when he had got over the shock, he tried to modify his behaviour both in the LHG and in his practice.

An effective understanding of the sources of power within an organisation, and how they play on the capacity of the players to confront unacceptable or deviant behaviour, is crucial, as the Case Studies A and C in Chapters 7 and 9 show.

In order to test the capacity of the practice to understand and deal with aggression and the exercise of power, answering the following questions may be useful:

- who exercises authority in the organisation?

- who has most influence?

- where are the sources of power and who controls them?

- are there opportunities to discuss the above openly with all players?

- what techniques does the organisation use to handle aggression?

Leadership and setting the direction

The delivery of a common philosophy and direction, and the exercise of power within an organisation such as a PCG or a general practice, may be directly related to the exercise of leadership within that organisation. Throughout the examples in Part 2 and intrinsic to the underlying issues identified in this chapter, is that of the place and delivery of the leadership role.

A great deal has been written about the nature and place of leadership (Kotter, 1990) and indeed the NHS has become somewhat obsessed by the need to develop and train 'leaders'. There may be some confusion around the fundamental question as to whether there is a need in the NHS for good local managers and management. It may be that in the current climate leadership comes rather from the politicians, the professional organisations and the NHS Executive (NHSE). Within practice organisations, however, and the new groupings of practices as PCGs, LHGs and LHCs, the role of leadership remains as crucial and little understood as it has been over the past 18 years.

Leadership and management are two distinct but complementary functions. They may occasionally be found within one person, but frequently they are not. Irrespective, it is important to note the difference and not confuse the two. Management is discussed in Chapter 4. Leadership is discussed here because it is essentially about setting the direction (not planning its implementation), developing a vision of the future with others, devising strategies to produce the change needed to achieve that future and then coping with that change. Leadership requires the gathering of a broad range of data and identifying patterns to produce visions and strategies. Moreover, the leader has then in Heifetz's words to 'engage people in confronting the challenge, adjusting their values, changing perspectives, and learning new habits' (Heifetz, 1997).

Leadership is not a remote activity but bedded in the here and now – it has to happen all the time, and may be carried out by different people in the same organisation at different times. It certainly draws strength from a comprehensive, informal network of relationships, often with people relating in an intuitive and empathetic way, rather than the more formal relationship to roles and positions that tends to come into play with management. As Kotter (1990) says 'A peacetime army can usually survive with good administration and management up and down the hierarchy, coupled with good leadership concentrated on the top. A wartime army needs competent leadership at all levels. No one has yet figured out how to manage people effectively into battle; they must be led.'

The concept of leadership is one that many professionals find difficult to discuss, and indeed nowadays the sort of 'over-the-top' type leadership is rare because people are generally more vocal, more aware of their own place in the organisation and unwilling to follow orders blindly. Teamworking and consensus decision making have reduced the amount of old-style leadership (see Chapter 5).

But nevertheless, the functions of leadership as described above are vital to the health of an organisation. The answer lies in recognising where such skills and attributes lie and that they may be possessed by an individual who is not at the top of the practice's hierarchy, as Example 17 shows.

Example 17

The Shaw Practice had three partners, with a highly competent, recently appointed practice manager. All three partners recognised that they were lacking the energy and commitment to move the practice forward to keep up with the other practices in their PCG. The practice manager was keen and experienced. She and the practice nurse were representatives on the relevant PCG working groups and the practice nurse hoped to be elected to the board.

The practice manager was a lively, strategic thinker, who did not get bogged down in the day-to-day management of the practice, but ensured that the systems were in place to make it work. She kept an eye on the national scene and 'scanned the horizon' to see what was happening and how to take advantage of changes to enhance the practice's interest. She chaired the local practice manager's group and was the regional secretary of the Institute of Health Management. Her networks, both formal and informal, were extensive. Without in any way changing the implied sub-ordinate relationship she had with the partners, it was she who ensured that the practice was always reviewing its long-term strategies and maintained its capacity to meet change with enthusiasm and success.

This is not a usual scenario (Jelley, 2000). Indeed, one of reasons there is, in general, such difficulty in general practice for practitioners to handle policy and strategic management is because of a cultural distaste for leadership concepts. Partnership agreements are usually very vague in the areas of personal responsibility and accountability. This situation is changing slowly as a result of the introduction of quality assurance and governance issues into general practice, but 'flat' management approaches, or an inability to exercise 'followship', will continue to dog the development of effective primary care organisations. Example 18 is a refreshing sign of change.

Example 18

The eldest partner in the Oldfield Surgery was about to retire. He had been a very reluctant senior partner and the remaining partners decided that they would establish an executive partner post (instead of using 'buggins' turn to become the senior partner). They drew up a job description, the prime attributes of which were:

- to be able to lead the practice into the 21st century
- to enthuse and encourage
- to help the practice to be courageous and approach change with fortitude instead of trepidation and reluctance.

> They recognised that what they were looking for was a leader and not someone to manage the practice. They had an effective practice manager to do that.
>
> They decided to hold a secret ballot. The by-now oldest partner was very keen to follow as senior partner and was reluctant to concur with the process. But he was persuaded. The youngest partner had been with the practice ten years and was a quiet, thoughtful but determined woman with clear ideas of where general practice was going, and was keen to place the practice in the vanguard of those developments. To her surprise and the delight of her colleagues in the partner ballot she was elected executive partner, and in the staff informal ballot she came top as well.

Many GPs and their colleagues are unsure of the future. The end of fundholding, the development of PCGs, LHGs and LHCs, the imminence of PCTs in England, the potential prospect of professional revalidation and likely changes in their love–hate relationship with the current system of continuing medical education (CME) all conspire to create uncertainty. From the GPs' perspective, practice survival on a day-to-day basis may take priority over educational and even organisational development initiatives (Carlisle *et al.*, 2000). In this, as every other period of change and threat, the need for the leadership function to be identified and appropriate steps taken to ensure it is fulfilled is essential. Leaders are comfortable with high risk and change. They are needed to help others through uncertainty and upheaval by keeping a clear view of the future (however near or far that view has to be), inspiring and encouraging, giving the framework within which everyone can manage the changes and implement the policies.

To test what leadership exists in a practice, the following questions are often asked:

- who is (are) the leader(s) in the organisation, and why are they seen as such?

- does the organisation need a leader and why?
- how is leadership demonstrated, what style is exercised?
- is there a clear job description for all the leadership roles?
- is there a 'power behind the throne', and if so why?
- does the organisation discuss its leadership?

Frequent recommendations arising from the issues of common philosophies and leadership

A number of common recommendations in relation to achieving a common philosophy and value system, as well as identifying the nature of leadership, arise at the end of a practice consultancy visit. They can be summarised as follows:

- make clear and explicit where the practice is going
- identify what contributions are expected from each member of the practice
- make clear and explicit what standard of performance is expected of each member of the practice
- clarify the nature of the leadership appropriate and necessary to deliver these.

4
Management awareness

Introduction

The capacity to establish and deliver decisions on common philosophies and values, as described in Chapter 3, is related directly to a second underlying issue. Chapter 4 addresses that second underlying issue; namely, the part played in practice by good management and the relevant competencies needed and available to discharge that part effectively. This is particularly true as the skills and experience required to handle the complex management issues that can arise in general practice organisations are often not covered in medical education and young doctors rarely get the chance to test their management aptitude and skills before becoming partners.

Apart from this lack of management skills training, other obstacles to management awareness include:

- the tendency for doctors to personalise issues as shown in Case Study A in Chapter 7, to adopt the 'doctor' rather than employer role and to confuse the caring advocacy of a health professional role with the firm directive role as manager. This can lead to mixed messages to staff and manipulation of the partners. This approach may also lead to staff being blamed for their mistakes or failures rather than praised for their success. It can be due to the inability or unwillingness of partners actually to recognise their own limitations and lack of management awareness. Frequently the mere spelling out of the legal and social consequences of poor management can bring about a realisation of the lack of appropriate knowledge and skills

- difficulties in partner decision making. This may be due to an unwillingness to spend time testing fully the consequences of a potential solution. A lack of clarity of roles and responsibilities among partners, as well as staff, can add to the underlying lack of confidence in the practice's management

- an unwillingness or inability to delegate effectively can be another cause of difficulty both for other partners and health professionals and for staff, particularly the practice manager

- the frequent under- or misuse of tools such as meetings and planning to help overcome these problems.

These issues are discussed in turn below.

Role awareness: the manager's responsibilities

Chapter 3 described the important role that leadership plays in ensuring an effective organisation. Management has an equally important and complementary role. Frequently in primary care the two roles are carried out by the same group – the partners and practice manager, or the PCG chair and chief executive. As stated earlier, there is often no clear understanding of the differences between them, and therefore of the considerations that are needed both to assess their effectiveness and to fill the gaps. Example 19 gives an instance of this.

Example 19

In a three-partner practice, the two senior partners, David and Jonathan, shared responsibility for the detailed day-to-day financial and staffing matters. They did all the hiring and firing, dealt with pay and kept the accounts with the help of an accounts clerk. The third partner, Michael, was not interested in practice management and left it all to them. The practice manager, Dawn, was highly frustrated as her job was largely to do the rotas under guidance, and manage the reception area and supplies. She was given no direction or framework within which to work, and so had to be very reactive. She was looking for another job as she felt undermined and demoralised, unable to manage the practice within a strategic framework provided by the partners.

At the end of the year the accountant announced that insufficient money had been put aside for the practice's tax bills. At the same time, one of the receptionists accused David of harassment. The two senior partners were so involved in the day-to-day management that they were unable to stand back and see this coming, or see the way out. Dawn put her advice in writing to David. In that letter she stated that in her view the steps that David was proposing to take, namely to summarily dismiss the receptionist for poor performance and unacceptable behaviour, would put the practice in breach of her contract of employment and be likely to land them before an employment tribunal. She explained that the lack of practice procedures in relation to equal opportunities, performance and discipline would tell against them, and that she would be happy to take on the task of dealing with the issue. What she needed from him and the other partners was the framework within which she would manage.

David had little insight into the problem or his part in it, and continued to handle both matters himself. As a result of his inexperience and lack of expertise in either personnel management or financial management, the practice was indeed taken to an employment tribunal and was required to reinstate the receptionist. Dawn found a new practice that allowed her to manage appropriately.

The accountant told them that they would have to cut back on their drawings by a third to meet the tax liabilities. That spurred the third partner into action and a new practice manager was employed on a very different basis, namely to run the financial and resource base of the practice, within boundaries set by the partner, but with delegated responsibilities to act within that framework.

Management is about coping with complexity. As Zaleznik (1977) states, 'Without a solid organisational framework even leaders with the most brilliant of ideas may spin their wheels . . .'.

In small organisations it may be that the manager must be the leader. However, it is still true and important to recognise that 'some people have the capacity to become excellent managers but not strong leaders. Others have great leadership potential but have difficulties becoming strong managers' (Kotter, 1990). Example 20 exemplifies this.

Example 20

A large, eight-partner practice had a sophisticated and complex management structure under the executive manager, who was a non-clinical partner. There were four assistant managers each handling one aspect of a complicated organisation that included dispensing and minor surgery, as well as managing some community services, such as chiropody and physiotherapy. The assistant managers were given a lot of autonomy to manage their areas within the policy framework set by the partnership. They were also expected to contribute to the development and review of the practice's policies, as well as head a significant team of often multi-skilled staff.

When a vacancy arose for the assistant manager (patient services), the partners advertised the post internally and three staff applied. The outstanding candidate was, they thought, the current head of reception, who had been with the practice for seven years, knew and applied the systems and procedures, and was liked and respected by all. She was thorough and a person for detail, had a good sense of humour, and was articulate and apparently confident.

When she was appointed, it became clear very quickly that she needed a lot of support and development in some elements of her new job, and that in particular she did not have a natural capacity to think strategically. Moreover, while she had been admired and liked as the head of the reception team, she was not able to inspire and motivate from outside that team. Her management skills were corrupted by her loss of confidence – and the organisation's – in her capabilities. She resigned after six months and the practice learned a very important lesson.

Management is often portrayed as boring and dull, unlike leadership, which is exciting and sexy. People who are inspirational and charismatic are leaders, while people with no imagination or capacity to take risks are managers. As usual, neither portrayal is true. The goals of management tend to arise out of necessity rather than imagination, they respond to need, and managerial culture will tend to emphasise rationality and control. But managers work with people and leaders often work alone.

There is a belief that management requires reflective, systematic planning, whereas in fact managers frequently work at an unrelenting pace, their activities characterised by brevity, variety and discontinuity. To manage often requires less than total information systems; often it is based on verbal communication, telephone calls and meetings over documents. Management is not a science or a profession but rather a series of activities based on judgement and intuition. The case studies in Part 3 demonstrate how lack of awareness of this concept of active management can lead people to believe that management is easy, and often they leave it to the newest and most inexperienced partner (as in Case Study A, Chapter 7).

In broad terms, the management tasks are to manage the interpersonal relationships within the organisation, to liaise with all and intervene as necessary to help people work effectively and supportively together. Part of this also is to represent the organisation both within and outside the organisation. The interaction with colleagues is important in order to pass on and obtain information, what Mintzberg (1980) calls 'the manager as the nerve centre of the organisation'.

To test the management capacity of the practice, answering the following questions may help to identify areas that need more work:

- has the management task within the organisation been discussed and described? If so, how and where?

- how is the management task delegated and to whom (if it is)?

- how are they equipped/skilled to do so now, and how do they keep up to date?

- how would you characterise the management style of the organisation?

- have you asked those working in the organisation if they find the style supportive or inhibiting?

- what processes do you have to deal with the latter answer?

- does the management style reflect your style? If not, how could you change it?

Decision making and problem solving

The most significant management tools are decisions, so how to make good decisions is a key skill for any organisation to foster and develop. There are many different decisions with different levels of importance, urgency and significance. As we have seen in Chapter 3, power is an important element in what makes an organisation tick. For many people the importance, urgency and significance of their decisions are direct measures of their power and a demonstration of it, and therefore the three elements are often overstated. Thus, it is important for the management team to analyse and identify the different nature of decisions before deciding on the most effective processes of decision making an organisation needs.

Day-to-day choices

There are decisions that are merely choices between several routes, framed by a clear overall policy. For instance, receptionists make decisions hourly about appointments, where and what to offer. These have to be instantaneous as the patient is on the phone or at the desk. A good framework agreed by all parties with areas of discretion stated and monitored means that access to the surgery for the patients can be smooth and as quick as possible. In contrast, if there is no agreed framework then receptionists will have to make decisions based on individual experience and preference, and the odds are that there will be a lack of consistency and equity in accessing surgery time across the patient population.

Resource decisions

Where there is an element of resource expenditure involved, as in money or time, it is still possible to set parameters, such as financial spending limits, within which individuals can exercise their individual decision-making skills. It is common to have a petty cash fund for instance, or to allow the practice manager to spend up to an agreed sum without seeking approval. Some organisations extend their options by imposing higher spending or decision-making limits to two or more partners or to a partner and the practice manager, for instance in relation to cheque signing.

Policy and framework decisions

Clearly, where a significant change is likely to result from decisions, be it in direction, resource use or relationships, the nature of the decision is significantly different and requires all parties to be involved, if not necessarily to agree. This would include decisions around key policy issues, such as fundholding, the purchase of a large piece of equipment, such as a computer system, taking on a new partner or practice manager, or deciding on priorities for the future.

In these decisions further clarification is invariably needed as to whether consensus decision making will be required, or majority decisions. If the latter, in what circumstances would that be acceptable? The means of arriving at such clarification relate very closely to the areas discussed in Chapter 3:

- do we have a common approach and philosophy?
- can we confront differences constructively?
- do we have someone who wields enough (but not too much) power to focus our discussions and help us face facts?

All these underline the need for open, trusting relationships.

What is a decision?

A decision is in essence a judgement, a choice between alternatives. It is rarely a choice between right and wrong. To make decisions about priorities it is important to be clear about what the options are. This requires full information about each project and the implications it may have for other activities and plans. Is the organisation able to deal with the implications of the decision? In Example 21, the implications of a decision were identified in time to prevent a disaster.

Example 21

Paul was a young and enthusiastic partner in a four-doctor practice on the outskirts of a new town. He was keen to become a trainer and urged his partners to allow him to put himself forward. The local scheme was very strict on its requirements and insisted on full practice compliance. So a separate consulting room for the registrar was needed and a practice library. The practice had neither.

Paul persuaded the partners that neither was a problem. The photocopier and files could be moved out of the storeroom and it could be turned into a small surgery, and the staff room could have a library at one end. The partners were dubious but agreed. Margaret, the most experienced partner, insisted, however, that as the practice manager and practice nurses would be closely involved in helping a registrar, they should be consulted. Paul was disappointed when the practice manager pointed out that the storeroom had no natural light and the registrar would need to share an examination room with Paul. There was insufficient room in the storeroom for a couch, a wash basin, a desk and two chairs, even assuming no children's toys or equipment. The nurse pointed out that the staff room was used for lunch and coffee breaks, that staff were relaxed and off duty at that time, and the atmosphere was, therefore, not conducive to reading or studying. Neither was against the idea but felt that before a decision was taken its full implications and effect needed to be explored, and all data collected. A range of options then might be put forward and costed.

Information on timescales and availability of cash is important. There is no point in putting energy into a scheme which the practice cannot afford for a number of years, when an apparently less important project could be got under way and completed at once, as Example 22 shows.

Example 22

The same practice decided to build an extension before applying for training status. They wanted to put cash aside for the next two years and then build. The staff were furious. The reception desk was small and pokey. There was no private area to discuss confidential matters, there was no room for the staff to sit down, there was insufficient room to lay out the appointment books and the telephone had to be on the wall, again breaching confidentiality.

The staff asked to see the doctors. They said that they had costed a redesign of the reception area that would cost less than a partner's monthly drawing, which would give them security and a little privacy and comfort, and give the patients more confidentiality. They asked if the doctors could revisit their decision to build an extension in order to become a training practice. They suggested extending the timescale from two years to three. The practice would thus be able to afford the front desk alterations immediately. The partners agreed.

The following questions help to focus on the key issues within this area:

- before making decisions does the management get all the information it can to inform that process, and if so, how?
- does the management act before all the information is collected, and if so in what circumstances?
- does the management scan the horizon and obtain information from outside the organisation?
- in what fora are decisions made, and are the parameters for those decisions clear?
- is everyone who should be, consulted and happy with the decision-making process in which they are involved? How would they change it?
- how does the organisation monitor the effectiveness of its management decisions?
- does the organisation record its decisions and analyse them annually for their appropriateness, timeliness and effectiveness?

Delegation

One of the commonest presenting problems for practices experiencing difficulties is that of time. Although this can often be addressed in some degree by better personal planning and prioritising, sooner or later it is essential to look at the ways in which effort is spread around the team — in other words, delegated. Indeed, the effort to schedule work better and to reduce involvement in routine activity may well sink under the weight of increasing workload, if proper planning and delegation do not take place.

The art is to plan ahead in most things. That is true of how and what to delegate. It is far better to anticipate increasing workloads and to develop positive systems to deal with them, rather than to assume 'something will turn up'. A critical point here is that delegation does not mean simply passing some of your work to others, either in a crisis or in an unplanned way. In the circumstances of most organisations in the health service today, delegation is 'the means of extending one's own competence by the competence of others, and the best delegation is to people who have skills beyond oneself' (Irvine and Irvine, 1996).

The inability to do this well and successfully has bedevilled the development of many practices. To some extent it relates to the ability to be clear about who does what and the accountability lines (*see* Chapter 6), and in relation to the ability of doctors to trust and therefore rely on others, including partners.

For partners in independent businesses, such as most general practices, delegating not only the responsibility for deciding on the action but delivering a particular part of the plan can cause difficulties. General practice is a flat management structure, often with a number of executive heads all on an equal footing. The way of dealing with this is to delegate within the partnership wherever possible, as well as to outside of it. This, of course, not only spreads the load but, if done well, can encourage people to develop and enhance skills and specialise as they would do clinically. Example 23 exemplifies this.

Example 23

The four-partner practice at Central Town was overwhelmed with work. The partners had high return consultation rates, the nurses were used largely for treatment and bloods, and the practice manager was used mostly as a senior receptionist. The doctors took the line that they, as partners, were the people liable at law for the practice. Moreover, they believed nurses took longer to triage patients than if the doctors had five-minute appointments interspersed with the largely ten-minute surgeries. They were determined to keep a close eye on the business side of the practice, as they had seen in their neighbouring practices what happened when doctors delegated too much, as they saw it, to a manager – loss of income and poor reputation for access. They worked on the principles that all decisions had to be unanimous, and all matters of staffing, finance and clinical standards had to be dealt with by all partners.

Although they recognised the impact of this on their stress levels and the way they were able to deal with patients – which was why they called in a diagnostic consultant – they were unable to see how to let go. They started by trying to give individual partners responsibility for key elements of the practice, with reporting back to the partners' meeting on how and what they had done in the partnership name. This was successful, particularly in relieving them of the need to know everything and be involved all the time. As a result they were able to reduce the partnership meetings to once a fortnight and to begin to have clinical meetings on alternate Fridays with the nurses and ancillary staff. This in turn led them to begin to delegate more to nurses and this relieved some of the surgery pressure. When their practice manager retired they were able to look at a role for the new practice manager, which included a large element of the practice day-to-day management being delegated to the new person.

Even more common, however, are those practices that believe they are delegating effectively, when in fact, they are failing to follow the rules. Consequently, they usually present with problems around the competence or effectiveness of colleagues to whom work has been delegated, without seeing that it is the nature of the delegation that is preventing the delegatee from having a chance to perform well. The first rule is to recognise that if someone fails to deliver a responsibility that you believe you have effectively delegated to him or her, their failure is yours.

First, in ensuring that as much as possible is delegated, look at the tasks that can be delegated. Broadly, there are three categories that can be given to others.

1 **Routine matters** that are also important to the patient's experience of the practice, such as deciding on the colour of the waiting room walls.

2 **Issues where other people's experiences and technical skills are greater**, such as in choosing a new computer system or operating a specialist clinic such as minor surgery.

3 **Tasks that others can do to free your own time**, for instance culling records or taking bloods.

Other people often see more of the game, so it is always worth asking others, particularly potential delegatees, if there is anything they think you could delegate effectively.

A clear analysis of how time is spent can reveal what falls into these three categories, what needs to be delegated, what ought to be delegated and what is feasible to be delegated. That does not mean that all the tasks so revealed *must* be delegated. It merely means clarity is needed about where the options for releasing time lie. The cost in overwhelming others may be too high, and so the reality of delegation may be that it puts more pressure on them to delegate it than to go on doing it.

As far as clarity is concerned, if the reasons for the delegation are not clear, then the person to whom the task is being delegated has little hope of understanding the reason for the delegation in the first place. To be successful, the purpose needs to be established, then the delegatees need to be told what tasks are involved, what is expected of them and what constitutes effective performance, as Example 24 illustrates.

Example 24

After going on a course, a partner decided to institute an HRT clinic. The other partners thought it was a good idea. She told one of the receptionists to put up a notice in the reception area indicating that one of the doctors specialised in HRT matters and giving the times when she was available. The receptionist did so and told the other receptionists to block off the partner's surgeries for those times to free her to see patients with HRT concerns. As there was not a great rush of patients the partner spent some hours twiddling her thumbs. She realised her mistake but blamed the receptionist for 'taking her literally'. The reception staff were upset at being blamed for the failure of an idea in which they had not been involved, and on which their views and advice on the best way to let patients know about it had not been sought.

If the whole job is said to be delegated then it is very important that no part is kept back, especially the most enjoyable part! If it is, and it comes to light later, it might indicate a lack of trust, as shown in Example 25.

Example 25

A practice decided to go out to tender for a new accountant. The practice manager was told to visit a number of firms, draw up a specification and select a short list of three to present to the partners. This she did over a three-week period, and she spent a lot of personal time investigating their backgrounds, talking to existing clients and talking through the specification with them.

When she came to arrange the dates for the final presentations, the partners decided to have it when she was away on holiday, and so she was excluded from the most interesting and important part of the task she had done so well.

Resources to carry it out should go with the task. It is important that there are adequate resources to carry out the task and that there is a plan to provide them in advance. Such resources may include training, giving experience or examining how the work fits with other work the individual is doing. Using non-jargon language, especially when the task being delegated is a technical one, is very important. All messages should be checked for understanding and, where possible, anything passed on by word of mouth should be reinforced in writing to ensure no misunderstanding.

Further, it is very important that the person to whom the task is being delegated knows and agrees with the arrangements and timescale for its control and how it is to be monitored. With the best will in the world there may be mistakes. An instinctive reaction is to believe that it could have been done quicker, more thoroughly, more effectively, more accurately by the person doing the delegating. This is unlikely, given that the delegation is for the right reason in the first place. Criticism in any circumstance, but particularly when someone is acting on behalf of someone else, should be done in private, not in the reception area in front of the patients, or in the staff room in front of colleagues. Above all, every part of the delegation process should be faultless before blaming others.

Finally, it is important to recognise that delegation is not 'dumping'. The final responsibility for a task cannot be delegated to others. You can only make them accountable to yourself for the effective delivery of something that it is your responsibility to see is carried out properly. Most doctors know that well in clinical situations. It is equally true in organisational matters. When areas of less than optimum performance are discovered in relation to, for instance, staff management, the favourite cry is 'We left that to the practice manager'. This is inappropriate if the practice manager is not well-versed in, for instance, employment law. It is the employer's responsibility to ensure their employees are trained and equipped to carry out those tasks delegated to them. Example 26 illustrates this.

Example 26

Oldchester Practice was in trouble. The reception staff were up in arms because they had not received the normal Christmas bonus, usually departmental store vouchers. The partners had decided that the rates of pay were now sufficiently competitive not to need the bonus to keep staff motivated. They did not realise that the staff saw the vouchers as a personal 'thank you' and a sign of appreciation from the partners, separate from their monthly pay.

As a result, one of the receptionists, whose husband was a union representative in his own firm, suggested that staff join a trades union, and furthermore claim breach of contract. The practice manager was not well-versed in employment law. She was not aware that because the vouchers had been given for some years they had become part of the employment contract. To suddenly stop them without negotiation could indeed constitute a breach of that contract.

The partners of course blamed the practice manager for not warning them, but they in turn had not ensured that she was personnel trained. She had made it clear to them that she would have preferred to take expert advice on the withholding of the vouchers beforehand. The partners decided to re-institute the bonus but the atmosphere was never the same, although the staff did not in fact join a union.

Box 4.1 sets out in summary the basic rules of delegation.

Box 4.1: Rules for good delegation

- Never do work that others can do.
- Ask others if they know of other areas that could be delegated.
- Always be clear about the purpose of the task or authority being delegated.
- Make sure that, wherever possible, the whole job is being delegated.
- Use clear and jargon-free language when delegating.
- If mistakes arise, criticise in private and constructively.
- Ensure the timescale and monitoring arrangements for the delegation are agreed with the delegatee.
- Recognise that final responsibility for the task cannot be delegated.
- Take advantage of any criticism that may come from delegation.

It is difficult to be accountable for the work of others, particularly if you are legally, professionally and ethically responsible for what that person does in your name. It is often this concern that prevents professionals from allowing colleagues enough freedom to enable them to use their initiative and thus achieve success.

Answering the following questions gives a good guide to the effectiveness of your practice's delegation skills.

- Have you explored whether there are things that you do that could be done another way – have you looked at the possibility?

- Are there things that you do that could be done as well by others in the team?

- Are there things that you do that could be done better by others in the team?

- When you delegate a task, do you always check the delegatee's understanding of why the task is needed?

- Do you delegate the authority needed to complete the task when you delegate it?

- Do you ensure that the delegatee has the resources to complete the task to your standard?

- Does the delegatee know what that standard is? How do you know?

- When did you last praise a delegatee? When did you last criticise him or her, either directly or indirectly, to a third party?

- Do you know if you can leave the person to whom you are delegating this task to get on with it alone, or do you need to check regularly, and have you negotiated this with them beforehand?

- If the latter, are you confident that you are seen as supporting, rather than interfering?

- If a delegatee makes a wrong decision, what do you do?

- Do you think that if you delegate too much you will have insufficient to do yourself?

Effective approaches: meetings

Decisions that cannot be delegated to a single person usually get taken at a meeting. Everyone groans about meetings — 'they are a nightmare' is the frequent cry. Often this is because they are not carefully thought out, their purpose agreed and clarified, the membership positively decided and the outcomes monitored. In other words, everyone who is there needs to know why they are present, what is expected of them, what the issue(s) is and what is decided. Box 4.2 gives a few ideas of what people use meetings for.

Box 4.2: Uses of meetings

- For entertainment.
- To make decisions.
- As a battle or duel.
- As an opportunity to take stock of a situation.
- To exchange information.
- As an assembly or place of worship.
- As a means of getting agreement of opposites in public.
- As a stage.

There are a number of simple rules that can fundamentally improve not only the effectiveness of meetings, but also the way people view them and therefore the effectiveness of the decisions that are taken.

A meeting needs a chair to hold court and keep the process under some kind of order. Nobody expects the chair to be a psychologist or counsellor, but the aim is to keep the meeting moving constructively forward towards a positive goal — a decision, an agreement or an illumination. It does not have to be the same person each time, but whoever it is should be someone who is respected and heeded by the rest.

Ideally, the chair should decide on the business of the meeting beforehand and ensure that it is communicated to those who must or could be present. Similarly, it is the chair's job to ensure that everyone knows what has been agreed and who is doing what, by when. Often someone who takes notes at the meeting does this work. Keeping a record is vital, if only of the agreed decisions. If the note taker is also the agenda maker and action chaser then they also need to be fairly senior in the pecking order. They need to be able to 'nag' constructively and insist on answers.

The agendas should be focused and timed. The order of proceedings is also important. Example 27 shows how it can be controlled.

Example 27

The practice meeting was at midday. As usual, three of the four partners were present, the practice manager, the senior practice nurse, the health visitor and the registrar. The practice manager was the clerk and drew up the agenda, which had been circulated beforehand. There were several important matters about the LHCC development and two recent government green papers to be discussed.

The chair was Jane, the middle partner. She suggested that they vary the order of the agenda to take one or two minor housekeeping matters first until John was able to join them for the meatier discussions. When John arrived two or three minutes later they were able to get on with the key items.

At the end of the hour, the chair asked if there were any other matters anyone wanted to raise which had not been thought of when the agenda was drawn up. The practice manager said that she had hoped that all would have completed their preference sheets for the Christmas and New Year rota but they had not, so reluctantly she was raising it at the meeting. She had produced a rota, which she proposed they adopt and if it did not fit with anyone's plans they should have the responsibility for changing with someone. It really was now too late to wait any longer.

Peter and John expostulated and demanded to know why she had not raised this at the beginning of the meeting. The answer was simple – if she had, they would have spent the entire meeting dealing with an issue

> which, though important, was now so urgent that there was little room for debate or argument. It would have been a waste of a meeting, and most importantly the issues that needed to be discussed would have been driven off the agenda. The meeting agreed the practice manager's suggestion and partners gave more thought to their returns to requests regarding rotas in future.

In terms of handling a meeting well, there are three main rules:

● **keep the group together**

Although there is a need to test arguments and 'bottom out' issues, the chair must try to ensure that argument does not become personal and people do not become backed into a corner.

● **keep the group focused on the subject in hand**

The chair needs to keep alert to stop known wafflers taking the group down blind allies, and to be firm in bringing the group back from an easy and comfortable discussion to tackling the really difficult question under discussion. One way of doing this is to reflect back all the time to the group what is being said and where they have got to in the discussion or argument, and check that everyone understands. This is where the chair can keep the discussion going forward by emphasising the positive aspects of the discussion.

● **protect the weaker members of the group**

There is a need to protect some members of the group from those who see meetings as an opportunity to exercise power and strut their stuff. The way of doing that is to ensure space and time is given when someone who is hesitant and slow indicates that they want to speak. Equally in checking understanding and agreement, it is often important to go round the table one by one.

Questions that are useful to ask in this area are set out below:

- do you have regular meetings with specific purposes?
- do you regularly review those meetings and purposes?
- do you regularly review the attendees?
- are the meetings chaired effectively, or does the chair need some training?
- do the meetings have agendas, and are they minuted?

Effective approaches: planning

> A group of soldiers in the First World War were lost in the Alps. One of them found an old crumpled map in the bottom of his kitbag. With relief the group followed the map to base camp. When they arrived, one of the officers looked at the map and told them that it was in fact a map of the Pyrenees.

Planning is not always about a written document — it can be a matter of confidence and belief.

One of the most important areas in which effective decision making is needed is in planning. Whereas leaders set the direction of the organisation, the management role is to plan. Setting the direction is not the same as planning; rather they complement each other. Without direction and an overall goal (*see* Chapter 3), plans tend to be short-term and ineffective, but no long-term strategy has any meaning if it cannot be translated into a tangible form, namely a plan that can determine action. As Kotter (1990) says, 'Companies manage complexity first by planning and budgeting — setting targets or goals for the future, establishing detailed steps for achieving those targets, and then allocating resources to accomplish those plans'.

Most practices have got used to producing a business plan each year for the health authority. For many it is a missed opportunity to reflect on the aims and direction in which the practice is travelling, and to reprioritise the ways of achieving the overall goal, as Example 28 shows.

Example 28

In a five-partner practice, one of the partners, Jim, was a stickler for detail and following up decisions. The other four were dreamers and ideas people, who found the day-to-day running of the practice rather tedious and uninteresting. They were happy to leave production of the annual business plan to Jim and the practice manager. The latter two spent hours producing very detailed plans with targets set for each component; names were attached to each target for delivery, with timescales for performance. They took it to the partnership meeting and it was agreed without discussion.

When Jim tried to get the partnership to review their achievement against the plan, he ran into great difficulties. The four partners who had not been involved discovered that the plan committed them to changing the way the computer was used to audit a range of services that were not their highest priorities, such as setting up a sports injury clinic. The practice manager was keen on this as he saw it as a way of increasing practice income. The plan did not include the development of a nursing policy to enable better use of the nurse practitioner or reflect the wish of the four partners to close the list to reduce pressure and enable them to move to longer consultation times.

Because they had not involved themselves in, and did not see the value of, the process Jim was trying to impose, they had agreed to a meaningless plan that four of them did not support and the fifth could not implement.

Case Study B in Chapter 8 shows a practice trying to get to grips with this by taking time out to assess where the practice was on its path towards its end goal, and to brainstorm what and how it might progress. It fed into that exercise the needs of the individuals and their personal aspirations, and contained it all by adding in resource constraint. The result was a realistic and achievable plan for progressing towards the common goal.

To do this effectively everyone needs to know what part of the plan is down to him or her, and be clear about everyone else's role. That of itself means effective delegation, in a way that enables the individual and the organisation to be clear.

The following questions are useful for the practice to consider in looking at the way it uses the tool of good planning:

- have we discussed the value of planning for the future, and if so what was the outcome and why?

- if targets have been set, are plans in place to ensure that there are resources and capacity to deliver them?

- if not, how are the aims and ambitions of the organisation to be achieved?

- what systems are in place to monitor whether the organisation is on target?

- does the organisation believe it has no control over its own destiny?

Frequent recommendations arising from the issues involved in management awareness

A number of common recommendations in relation to enhancing management awareness arise at the end of a practice consultancy visit. These recommendations can be summarised as follows:

- to recognise limitations in relation to management skills
- to restructure and review decision-making processes
- to develop means of planning ahead and allocating tasks and roles to others
- to delegate effectively.

5
Working across boundaries

Introduction: teamwork not tribalism

In earlier chapters, much reference has been made to people working together in various ways. Indeed, poor teamworking is often an unrecognised underlying problem that has been identified throughout the consultancy visits. Chapter 5 tackles the obstacles to and ways forward for working across professional, attitudinal and physical boundaries.

Although much effort — and some might say lip service — has been put into teamworking within primary care teams, our experience shows little evidence that it has improved significantly. Indeed, more recent experience of visiting practices suggests that professional groups have tended to move back into their professional shells to protect their specialism, rather than venture further to see what it is like to work with others who may be tackling the same professional areas of patient care. This can confuse patients and reduce their confidence. And it is the complete antithesis of clinical governance focused on clinical teams that are expected to accept some collective responsibility for service delivery and performance.

Examples of this retreat include the enhanced role of nurses in one-to-one situations with patients (nurse practitioners, health promotion nurses and so on). This carries the danger of increasing their isolation rather than their involvement with the health team. Throughout the health system time and pressures of workload have reduced the informal and social interactions that are the glue to a multiprofessional team approach to patient care. This is compounded by the use of the term 'professional' to relate to clinical staff (usually doctors and nurses), implying as it does that non-clinical staff are unprofessional.

Inadequate people management lies behind the lack of performance and poor morale that is often present in a practice, and it underlies a lot of the issues around interpersonal behaviour. Selecting the right people to work within the practice, where it is possible to do so, is a vital component of this. However, employment procedures are generally not well thought through in practice. Even where there is a practice manager in post there are many examples of selection and recruitment being carried out with hearts rather than heads, often influenced by the pressures of time. Knowledge of the changing framework of employment rights and employer obligations is often scanty, particularly on human rights, harassment, full- and part-time working, sickness and pension, maternity and parental rights, and so on.

Our experience gives evidence that general practices are ill-equipped to deal with this agenda. Although human resource management is not the subject of this book, in discussing the underlying issue of how to work effectively with other people, some comment needs to be made on the employment framework. Chapter 3 referred to stress and bullying issues and treatment during employment, and Chapter 6 discusses the statutory duty of quality. Chapter 5 deals with the fair and due process of entry and exit from the practice, and matters of training and continuing professional development (CPD).

Often personnel management failings can be the symptoms of dysfunctional partnerships and teams already described in Chapters 3 and 4. Sometimes it is due to lack of insight into why people work. Frequently, staff and partner morale problems have at their root a failure by partners to appreciate the different motivational forces at work in a team, and how to energise them. Only by doing so can a practice handle all the change that surrounds working in the NHS today and for the future.

The pros and cons of teams

In the 1950s, a commercial plane set off from Tulsa. After an hour's flying, there was a tap at the cockpit door. One of the passengers asked the pilot how to work the coffee machine, as there were no cabin staff. The pilots had left without checking that the stewards and stewardesses were on board – they were not seen as part of the plane's crew.

Teams are people doing something together. As Robbins and Finlay (1997) say, 'The *something* that a team does isn't what makes it a team; the *together* part is.' All GPs work in teams (RCGP, 1999) – even single-handed ones have reception and nursing staff. Early government White Papers (*Choices and Opportunities*, DoH 1996a; *A Service With Ambition*, DoH 1996b) challenged the traditional values of a doctor- and illness-centred service, redefining the primary healthcare team and placing users and public health as its paramount concern. Further, the 1997 White Paper (*The New NHS: modern, dependable*) set out statutory obligations for multiprofessional PCGs to ensure quality services. Although GPs are still placed in the senior managerial level within each locality, the emphasis is on working in partnership.

A good example of working well across boundaries is given in Example 29.

Example 29

A practice in the heart of London was large. It consisted of seven partners, four practice nurses, two counsellors, two interpreters, three attached social workers, a visiting nutritionist, a practice manager, an assistant practice manager, a senior receptionist and a full receptionist team, three secretaries, a computer operator and a full complement of attached nurses. It was clear to them all that only full multidisciplinary teamworking would ensure that such a large and complex organisation worked in a way that not only delivered a good service, but also gave satisfaction to all.

The day-to-day working of the practice was delegated to the practice manager and her assistant, and she was supported by each of the partners having a specific area of interest in the management of the practice. The partners all recognised that it was vital to have everybody on board when looking at new developments. These included:

- enlarging the premises
- attracting consultants to run clinics at the surgery
- dealing with the demands of the PCG for better data
- developing nurse triage services
- integrating with the new out-of-hours services and NHS Direct
- developing more effective appraisals for all
- ensuring they were meeting the demands of the new clinical governance papers.

To achieve some kind of priority listing for all these activities, they held a practice meeting with all the members of the practice. They shut the practice for a half-day, having given due notice to patients, and employed a retired receptionist and locum doctor to deal with emergencies.

At the meeting everyone had their say and agreed a list of priorities. Everyone was then asked to sign up to a series of working groups set up to design and implement these top priorities, at the top of which were the extension of the premises, the nurse triage and clinical governance.

The premises team attracted 20 volunteers and it was clear at the first meeting that there were far too many people involved. As there were so many elements within the one big project they decided to set up a steering group and a series of small teams dealing with specific aspects, such as finance, space needs, income generation opportunities, patient involvement, interior design and fittings, and so on. Each of these groups had a representative on the steering group, which was the body that liaised most closely with the architect and the health authority.

The teams included a wide range of skills and backgrounds, and everyone tended to forget what the individual team members did in their day jobs when they were working in the team. Often the meetings were out of hours, at people's homes, frequently followed by a meal. When the work was done each project team disbanded.

There were few instances of conflict and when the premises were opened everyone agreed that the whole process had been a very good

> example of using teamwork to get a project completed effectively. More importantly, hidden talents had been revealed or created, which would be of use in the future. They decided to use the same approach for the nurse triage project, though in a smaller way, and then to develop the clinical governance priority.

Teams and team-building, while not the panacea of all ills they were thought to be some years ago, are needed to ensure consistency and common practice, as well as safety and quality, between individuals and groups and to deliver the aspirations of the organisation. They are particularly important in resolving tensions between administrative and financial efficiency and clinical efficacy. Moreover, as old hierarchical structures under a senior partner disappear, the need for cohesion is greater to ensure that individuals fulfil their potential through consolidating team developments.

The classic reasons for supporting the concept and practice of teams are set out in Box 5.1.

Box 5.1: Why teams work

- Teams increase productivity.
- Teams improve communications.
- Teams are able to do work that individuals or single disciplinary groups cannot.
- Teams make better use of resources because they help focus ideas.
- Teams are more creative and better at problem solving, mainly because they combine multiple perspectives and tend to be motivated to find solutions.
- Teams tend to make better decisions because of the shared knowledge.
- Teams mean better services, again because of increased knowledge.
- Teams mean improved processes because they help break down boundaries.
- Teams help stability within an organisation.
- Teams help ensure the right leaders emerge, ones that command the greatest support or are accepted most easily by the team.

The reason why teamworking is so important lies in the fact that when relationships among team members break down, the effect on the care that patients receive is highly deleterious. Patients suffer, either directly or indirectly, as resources are squandered and duplicated. In contrast, patient care is enhanced when there is good teamworking, so there is a need to monitor and improve the way teams function. And this concern with the wellbeing of the patient is the centre of all team goals.

As stated earlier, it is also important to recognise that team-working is not the answer to all evils and, indeed, the wrong team doing the wrong task in the wrong way can be a very destructive force. Case Study A in Chapter 7 shows what can happen if teams become too insular and inward looking. There may be confused goals and objectives within teams, and bad leadership and personality conflicts. This may mean bad decisions that are harder to reverse or disentangle because they carry the authority of a team decision.

Primary care has evolved steadily from a uniprofessionally led service to today's multiprofessional teams, which increasingly provide comprehensive care within the community. Despite this greater team approach and integrated care within the community, general practice still has a lot to learn about how to demonstrate valuing people, to delegate effectively, to select and monitor supportively the work of others, and to recognise the value of team learning.

The pressure on the medical profession to become more involved as team players in the delivery of healthcare has increased over the past 20 years. General practice has been slow to respond, partly because every additional team player is a member of the payroll, partly because the nature of general practice is just that – generalist and individualistic – making initial decisions about all problems that patients bring. Lack of specificity and an inability to define the job are fine when things are going well, but once challenges appear in terms of other potential suppliers of the skill and expertise, then the lack of a job description is a source of anxiety. Over the past 20 years other professionals have taken new powers and responsibility for patient treatment and the proposals within the government's NHS Plan will enhance this (DoH, 2000). It is important to ensure that in itself this does not lead to a 'dog in the manger' attitude on all sides.

Developing understanding across team boundaries

There are three real ways in which a practice can build a team. The first is by encouraging exchange of information and knowledge across boundaries. The team that learns together plays together is an old adage (adapted) but true. So much of the suspicion and aggression in teams is due to ignorance and assumption about the relative value and the role of other members of the team. Taking time out to educate each other in all the activities that go to make up the delivery of general practice can bring incalculable benefits, as shown in Case Study A and Example 30.

Example 30

The new practice nurse in a busy urban practice was overwhelmed with her treatment clinic load. She emerged from her surgery, fully gloved up, and shouted in the general direction of the reception area for some forms that she needed urgently to give to the patient she was treating.

The receptionists were very busy handling patients at the desk booking appointments, on the phone to other patients trying to book appointments, dealing with the doctors doing surgery calling for patients to come through and taking lab reports being phoned through. They all ignored her.

Ten minutes later she got the forms herself and told the senior receptionist she would be reporting the matter to the partners and 'something would have to be done'. The receptionists were incensed, the nurses were angry and the doctors were irritated. At the next practice meeting the matter was raised and everyone became very heated about who was busier than whom and whether clinicians had a higher rating in the practice than others. It became clear that no one understood the roles of the different parties or how their activities affected each other. The practice manager suggested that, on a regular basis, each professional group present to the rest of the practice their role and their perceptions of what the rest of the practice could do to make their lives easier.

The exercise was very illuminating and it became clear that patients were the most important people, so everyone dealing with them directly – be they receptionists, nurses or doctors – had the top priority in terms of everyone else's support. A judgement had to be made by each as to whether dealing with an anxious patient on the phone took higher precedence at that particular moment than a patient who was in a hurry to have their travel injections completed. Understanding and empathy were the name of the game.

A second way is through continuing professional development (CPD), a process of lifelong learning for all, to meet the needs of patients and deliver NHS priorities. CPD must focus on the needs of patients, be a partnership between individuals and the organisation, and meet individual career aspirations and learning needs. Although primary care professionals probably have better opportunities for postgraduate learning than other NHS colleagues, there are still huge shortcomings in the present system. These include insufficient and wrongly targeted resources, inappropriate learning methods and difficulties in delivering integrated learning (CMO, May 1998).

The content of courses, and consequently learning, is often inappropriate for multiprofessional learning. However, better opportunities exist through external validation such as Investors in People (IIP), RCGP, Fellowship by Assessment (FbA) and Quality Practice Award (QPA). All these give opportunities for shared learning and activity towards a common end, which is a good way to build a team.

Also, the practice professional development plan (PPDP) is a formalised way of developing the concept of the 'whole practice' as a human resource for healthcare, resembling the health promotion plan in general practice and increasing involvement in the quality development of practices. Case Study B in Chapter 8 is an example of how such an approach can work.

Above all, if individuals are provided with autonomy and a climate of equity and mutual respect between professionals is created, then a multiprofessional group will develop its own way of working and learning effectively together.

There are of course more traditional team-building activities in practices. Often focusing around a project can provide such a tool, as shown in Example 31.

Example 31

A practice had an extremely old computer system that was irritating everyone and creating bad feeling in an otherwise friendly and happy team. The senior receptionist felt particularly strongly that the issue should be grasped. She and one of the nurses put forward the proposal that a cross-boundary team should be set up to examine the use of the computer made by the practice, how other practices used theirs and what could be done to bridge the gap without huge expense. The partners were delighted and one of them agreed to join the working group, as did one of the community nurses who had a brother-in-law 'in computers', and another receptionist who had come from an acute hospital and had some experience of more sophisticated systems.

The steering group visited five practices, read the literature and visited three providers. They kept everyone informed of what was happening both at the monthly practice meeting and by individual briefing back in their own professional group. A report was brought at the practice meeting and then to the partners' financial meeting and the proposal to have presentations to the whole team were accepted

Apart from improving the use of the computer in the practice, the atmosphere and attitude of the members of the team were transformed

> with a clearer idea of their purpose and function. The members of the steering group in particular were focused on the project in hand and formed a strong bond. Even when the group was disbanded they retained camaraderie for some years afterwards.

There are many small tips that can help the team-building process and these are set out in Box 5.2.

Box 5.2: Team-building tips

- Only create teams when there is a clear purpose or task.
- Keep it small.
- Have a defined lifespan with a date for reviewing its effectiveness and achievement.
- Have a respected and energetic chair.
- Have clearly agreed modes of working and decision making.
- Understand and respect colleagues' personalities and motivations.

The following questions might help practices work out their approach to teams:

- have you actively discussed the benefits of teamworking in your practice?

- are the purposes of each team clear to all in the team and those outside it?

- are the reasons for each team and their purpose reviewed regularly?

- is the membership of each team reviewed regularly?

- are the team members from different professional groups within the practice?

- are there opportunities for multiprofessional learning?

- does the practice have a culture of praise rather than blame?

- are there appropriate and successful social relations within the practice?

Choosing the right team

Getting the right team members is of course crucial, be it partner or staff. The balance of skill, personality and fitness for the purpose is fundamental, as shown in Example 32.

Example 32

Ian was the driving force of a partnership of five. He attracted lively new partners, in particular Graham, who was another dynamic personality. Ian had a lot of outside interests. He was active in the RCGP and was nationally involved with audit and education. As a result, the practice was frequently in the vanguard of developments and acted as a pilot for experimental schemes on many occasions. Graham was developing the same interests, and the other partners were happy to reflect in the glory and enjoy the challenges, although they were less keen on the workload implications.

Graham decided at the age of 40 to change his career and go into full-time academic practice. This was a great blow to Ian, who had seen him as his successor in the driving seat of the practice. The other partners were less unhappy. They saw replacing Graham as an opportunity to bring in another quieter and more reflective partner, and create what they saw as a period of stability. They selected Kenneth against Ian's vote.

Ian retired five years later and the partners found themselves with no activist or much in the way of pragmatist. They appointed another reflective type of personality to replace Ian, without considering the shape of the team and where the drive and energy for handling the challenges of the future would come from. As a result the practice stagnated and staff became bored and frustrated.

The selection of partners and staff is a risky business, and people are often chosen on gut feelings and subjective criteria. Our experience is that, over the years, GPs have been resistant to ensuring that the whole process is carried out professionally and objectively. The concept of the practice as an informal, friendly, family group dies hard for good reason. But this does produce resistance to formalisation and preparation for bringing in new team members. A good example is given in Example 33.

Example 33

The appointment of the new practice nurse was a mistake. She was clinically competent but had little understanding of her own limitations and came across as arrogant and intolerant to the rest of the team. She ruffled feathers, including patients'.

The partners talked about what had gone wrong with her appointment as it had been a unanimous decision of the interviewing panel. One partner had been on holiday, another had been sick, so in fact only three of the five partners had been present and the practice manager had been at a PCG meeting. They had no external advice from an experienced practice nurse and the other members of the nursing team did not meet her. They agreed that they had asked her technical clinical questions only and had not tested her team qualities.

The nurse resigned and the practice learnt from its mistakes. They drafted possible questions for the interviews beforehand, using little scenarios to test the candidates' responses to team issues. They asked a local nurse practitioner to act as an external assessor. They ensured that the practice manager could be present and invited all candidates to visit the practice and meet the whole team before the interview. They asked team members to feed back comments to the practice manager. This time they appointed someone whose skills and clinical professionalism were undoubted but who also appeared to have a value system and approach that harmonised with the rest of the nursing team, and with the aspirations of the practice. She settled well and quickly, and also was able to introduce change and improvement.

Details of what constitutes a good selection process can be found elsewhere (Haman and Irvine, 2000), but some key tips are set out in Box 5.3.

Box 5.3: Recruitment tips

- Update job descriptions and include performance measures where possible.
- Spend time preparing the person specification.
- Allocate areas of questioning to interviewers.
- Use the interview as an opportunity to swap information.
- Compare each candidate with the job description and person specification.
- Decide after each candidate has been interviewed if they are fit for the job.
- Do not compare candidates with each other, unless you have more than one who you have decided can do the job as you wish.

Rarely do the interviewers have training and this recommendation is probably a counsel of perfection. However, the problems of facing the failures of any interviewing panel to address basic equal opportunities need to be borne in mind when interviewing.

De-selection is also important for the health of the groups and the practice. Again GPs, as we have seen, are not good at confronting poor performance in others, particularly long-serving or strong-minded staff, or partners. One incident is given in Example 34.

Example 34

A practice manager of seven years' standing had a major personal crisis and the partners were very sympathetic and understanding. When she returned to work she was much less committed and generally 'off the boil'. The finances of the practice, which she had handled brilliantly, were beginning to suffer. The partners did not feel able to talk to her about this, as she was, they thought, still fragile. So one of the partners offered to help her with the finances, an offer she accepted with alacrity. He effectively took it over.

After three more years of continual dissatisfaction and less and less commitment from her, the partners felt they could no longer let her deal with staff directly as she was causing upset. So they suggested that she should have a deputy to help with her workload. Again she accepted with alacrity.

Another year passed and she needed to have a hysterectomy. The partners immediately went into doctor mode and told her to take as long as she needed. When she went off, having had three months to plan for it, there was no provision made to back up her work. They could not access the finance software as she was the only one who knew the new password, she had changed the keypad number on her office door without informing anyone and her in-tray, when they got to it, was piled with unanswered letters and enquiries. They had kept no written records of the previous difficulties and behaviours they had experienced with her and felt unable to confront her while she was ill. The rest of the staff were either fed up because they had to take on the extra workload caused by this, or were surprised at how lenient and compliant their employers were. Behaviour and standards generally dropped, with staff coming in late, refusing to wear their badges, and nurses deciding their own clinics and hours of work.

Details of the technical processes involved with redundancy, redeployment and dismissal are the subject of a separate book (Haman and Irvine, 2001) but here it is important to point out that the relationship between an open and fair process of discipline and handling poor or inadequate performance is vital in maintaining a happy and well-motivated team. It is a frequently discovered, painful truth that it is occasionally better to be cruel to be kind. Failing to state problems clearly as they arise, with a constructive approach to preventing the incident happening again or developing a skill that is obviously missing, merely puts off the evil day. And that day will be more evil because the person concerned will have no knowledge of their failings in the past. Moreover, other staff and colleagues, seeing what behaviours and standards are apparently tolerated and condoned will use this as a model for their own behaviours and standards, as shown in Example 34.

Useful questions to be asked in relation to the selection of staff are as follows:

- are there up-to-date job descriptions for all the responsibilities in your practice?

- before a selection process takes place do you decide what sort of person you need, with what sort of skills and attributes?

- do you decide on suitability for a post against the job description and person specification, or do you change either to fit the candidate you like?

- do you use an external assessor to help in the interview process?

- do you have someone in the practice who is familiar and up-to-date with employment and equal opportunities legislation?

- do you have written disciplinary and grievance procedures?

Motivating others

Often doctors quite rightly complain about poor management of themselves by governments and the NHS. They need to reflect on the impact that de-motivating activity and negative criticism, when it comes without the supportive constructive criticism and recognition of what is good about the service, has on them. Sometimes reflecting in this way would help them to see how important good motivation is in developing and maintaining a good team in the practice.

The starting point is always to understand that different people work for different reasons and do the particular job they have for yet more varied reasons. These are often divided into what Hertzberg (1966) some years ago called *hygiene* and *motivating* factors. Box 5.4 sets them out, but in essence they are those factors which meet basic needs — avoiding pain from the environment and including drives such as hunger – and those which are more sophisticated and complex, and consequently likely to be present in different combinations in people.

Box 5.4: Hygiene and motivating factors

Hygiene factors
- Organisational policy.
- Administration.
- Supervision.
- Interpersonal relationships.
- Working conditions.
- Salary, status and security.

Motivating factors
- Achievement.
- Recognition for achievement.
- The work itself.
- Responsibility.
- Growth or advancement.

It is the motivating factors that are the primary cause of satisfaction and it is therefore very important to recognise that the provision of hygiene factors upon which many employers concentrate is insufficient to produce job satisfaction, as shown in Example 35.

Example 35

The partners organised a Christmas lunch for the staff three weeks before Christmas. They asked a drug company to sponsor it. They were surprised when only three staff of 24 accepted the invitation.

The next year they asked the staff what they would like to do. They offered to fund a dinner. The staff said they would prefer a buffet supper and disco. The partners agreed and all staff turned up, and funded their spouses to attend.

A second example shows another approach.

Example 36

A large fundholding practice assigned £10 000 from savings to establish a practice educational fund. This fund, administered by the partner responsible for training, was to be used to help members of the practice pay for educational activities which were deemed to be furthering the objectives of the practice, and which could not be supported from other sources. Examples of practice educational activities supported in this way included:

- one partner attending a diploma course in therapeutics in order to take overall responsibility for practice prescribing
- two partners strengthening their management skills, one by joining an MBA course and the other an Open University course in health services management
- a trainee practice nurse practitioner undertaking an honours degree for nurse practitioners
- the practice manager undertaking a diploma course in business administration
- a receptionist attending a new skills course
- an enrolled nurse on a conversion course to become an RGN
- a health visitor on study leave to develop skills in health needs assessment.

As a result all members of the ream felt fulfilled and valued.

One of the real problems about motivation in general practice is the complex role that doctors play in the surgery – they are owners and employers, as well as the coalface workers. Their support teams – the reception, nursing and administrative teams – would ideally need to supervise the clinician's work to be maximally motivated and to ensure optimum use of resources. This is clearly not possible because of the employer/ employee relationship with the doctors as partners/employers.

Motivation and inspiration energise people by satisfying the basic human need for achievement, a sense of belonging, a feeling of control over one's life. Good leaders motivate in a variety of ways — they articulate the organisation's vision, they involve people in achieving the vision, they support employees by encouraging, coaching and feedback, and role-modelling, and they recognise and reward success. Indeed, this exemplifies the fact that managing is not a series of mechanical tasks but a set of human interactions (Teal, 1996). These are all the more important when in a period of continuous change.

Before turning to that, here are some questions to test the motivational awareness of the practice.

- Do you know why your medical partners became doctors?

- Do you know what attracted the various members of your staff to your practice?

- Do the staff feel valued and respected? How do you know?

- Are members of the team encouraged to put forward ideas and suggestions, and do they get feedback on them?

- Are nurses in the practice differentiated from non-clinical members of the team in the way that they are treated by the partners?

Making effective changes

Over the past 20 years and for the foreseeable future there has been and will continue to be a tendency towards almost continual change, which in turn requires less rigid organisational structures, less reliance on traditional methods, and more flexibility and innovation. As Robbins and Finlay (1997) put it,

'We are passing through an official era of reinvention, re-engineering and transformation ... Change is pain, even when self-administered.'

The handling of change is an area that challenges managers, including GPs, most severely, even recognising that all management is about trying to achieve change with as little conflict as possible. The problem is that most people like things to remain as stable and familiar as possible. Resistance to change is born of fear, which is expressed as anxiety. Handling that anxiety and harnessing the energy it creates are major tasks.

The art is to retain the best of the old values or working practices, while providing a positive vision of the future. The aim is to reduce uncertainty by active communication and careful planning. One of the worrying lessons from the past is that there is an alarming ignorance of NHS changes and their implications in general practice, from the days of the New Contract (DoH, 1990), through fundholding, and now with PCG/PCT development. Working in localities, creating an effective governing body for new PCGs/PCTs, identifying local health needs and promoting public involvement will require major changes in the general practice way of working, even for those who have been in the forefront of change (Marks and Hunter, 1998).

The underlying issues around presenting problems in coping with change in general practice will include attitudinal inflexibility as well as fear of loss. In a group of people, be they partners or the whole practice, reaction to those problems will vary. Some will handle a lot of change well – the phrase is that they 'thrive on it'. Some will say they want it if only they had the resources to do it, but are unwilling to make do and find untapped resources or skills to help. Others feel bereft and alone, and are unable to share for fear of seeming uncommitted. If any of these sensitivities are handled badly the whole team can dissolve. For instance, if someone who takes time to absorb change is pushed too fast they will resist all the harder. Box 5.5 sets out the causes of resistance.

Box 5.5: Causes of resistance to change

- Fear of the unknown.
- Fear of failure.
- Fear of disruption.
- Fear of being left behind.
- Fear of not coping with the new.
- Fear of conflict.
- Fear of changed values and philosophies.
- Fear of surprise.

The effective manager deals with all these fears in all the players. First of all, everyone has to understand why there needs to be change and feel involved in bringing it about. Involvement is the best way of removing resistance at this early stage, and the advantage is that those involved will help each other come to terms with their difficulties.

It is also important to make change in a step-wise progression if possible, providing opportunities for amending plans if necessary. This of itself will instil confidence in the fainter-hearted.

Box 5.6 sets out some rules for good change management.

Box 5.6: Rules for good change management

- Plan and collate the information and facts needed.
- Involve others in the process.
- Communicate what you are planning to others with a stake in the outcome – and give the same message to all.
- Take negativity and cynicism seriously and discuss it openly.
- State the outcomes of the change, but leave choices within the overall decision.
- Create networks of those who can influence and support the change.
- Keep the impetus going, but minimise surprise – give advance warning.
- Follow through changes as they happen.

- Be prepared for mistakes and how to deal with them.
- Keep it simple.
- Recognise and compensate people for the extra time and energy involved in delivering change.
- Evaluate the change.

Ask yourself the following questions:

- what pace of change am I asking my organisation to tolerate?

- do I know who the innovators are in the practice?

- have I explained what I am trying to achieve?

- does the practice have a culture of supporting those who find change threatening?

- is this an organisation that listens to its team members?

Frequent recommendations arising from issues around working across boundaries

The most frequent recommendations made for improving this aspect of care have been as follows:

- improve people management through developing good employment practices to develop a culture that enables people to:
  - appropriately confront deviant behaviour
  - identify and depersonalise issues
  - develop a culture of review and revising standards upwards
- improve communications and the development of a culture of review and revising standards upwards

- provide more and better development and training in:
  - effective decision making
  - assertiveness
  - chairmanship
  - employment law
  - appraisal
  - financial management
  - quality assurance and audit
  - handling complaints
  - risk management
- create a culture of respect and effective communication.

6
Accountability to self and others

The nature of accountability

The three main underlying themes discussed so far – having common values and philosophies, being aware of the management needs of an organisation and working across boundaries – link with accountability, our fourth major underlying cause of difficulty for general practice. In common with all doctors, GPs have always been accountable – it is the extent and nature of that accountability that is changing (RCGP, 2000a). Until 20 years ago accountability in professions was largely limited to dealing with unethical behaviour in any members that might undermine the reputation and standing of the club. Trust and professional conscience largely regulated clinical practice, although breaches of terms of service could trigger action. Concern to take account of the concepts of quality and accountability in the eyes of the public was not common. Example 37 illustrates something of this, taken as it is from one of the earliest practice visits carried out.

Example 37

In 1984, Leadtown Practice was the only surgery in a small market town. The three partners were well-respected and active members of the community, being accorded status and authority in whatever part of the town's life they involved themselves. They opened the surgery at

> 9.00 am and closed it at 6.00 pm. They ran open surgeries on two mornings and had five-minute booked appointments at all other times. The premises were small, with a cramped waiting room, wooden benches for seating and no children's play area.
>
> The doctors were frequently late for surgery — a wait of 30 minutes or more for the surgery to open was not uncommon. There was no shelter in which the patients could wait — they stood in an orderly queue outside in all weathers.

This situation was tenable while public expectation was low and trust was high. The changing societal demands for explanation and certainty, together with a far lower threshold for tolerating error, have largely, though not entirely, put paid to all this. A whole raft of changes has both reflected a failure of public confidence in self-regulation and is a response to it. The changes include primary care and patient support groups, special interest and patient participation groups, together with an increase in successful litigation, a more aggressively controlling parliamentary style and the recognition by the media that tragic medical stories make better copy than good outcomes. These developments have revealed gaping holes in medical accountability, especially in general practice where the independent contract is one of the last areas of uncontrolled health expenditure and thus a prime target for any government with a need to meet ever-rising potential for improving the quality of life. It has thrown into relief the resistance of many GPs to invest time and money in describing what they do in a way that others — peers and lay — can test against a norm. The screw has been turned over the years and the amount of audit and quality review carried out has increased, although the quality of that work itself remains variable. It remains, in our experience, one of the single most limiting causes of practice stagnation or tension, as lack of data can undermine almost every aspect of clinical and organisational life.

However, in reflecting on this underlying cause for concern, it has to be borne in mind that the internal drivers for quality and sense of accountability that inform and guide most professionals are an essential platform for any effective and meaningful regulation, both managerial and professional. Changes or recommendations for action, both in individual general practices and more widely, must not damage personal desire for quality. Performance indicators are only measures of the measurable. They cannot measure commitment and that sense of conscientiousness on which quality for patients depends. Nor do they reflect the context of care. Employment contracts and the clinical governance enforced through those contracts are blunt instruments for ensuring accountability and quality without reducing the range and quality of care that is motivated by personal and professional pride and sense of responsibility (Example 38).

Example 38

Tregowan Medical Centre had six partners and two salaried assistants. The assistants worked three sessions each per week and delivered an acceptable quality of care. There were no patient complaints, and the staff found them generally amenable and hard working. However, they were not available to do any extras and declined to see patients after their allotted sessions. They did not attend practice meetings because they were not contracted to do so and they were held at lunchtimes. Although invited, they did not attend partnership meetings because they were held in the evenings. Consequently, the partners found themselves having to issue written bulletins on any changes in practice that came out of their meetings and discussions to ensure the assistants knew what was going on.

Nevertheless, the assistants felt second-class citizens and complained about being uninformed, but they were anxious not to get sucked into all sorts of activities and practices for which they were not paid. The staff were irritated by assistants who said no to seeing extra patients and the partners were confused by doctors who 'worked to contract'. When both assistants became pregnant and left, a full partner was appointed.

The underlying issue around accountability will be emphasised further as professional revalidation and managerial clinical governance and its components – audit, risk management, education, complaints and quality assurance – take effect.

Chapter 6 offers some reflections on the key areas that appear to cause most difficulty for practices in changing their approach to quality and accountability. It starts with audit – knowing what you are doing against standards agreed beforehand. This has had a mixed history and the translation of that into quality assurance even more so. The major tools for both are performance monitoring, of which appraisal based on the areas of practice described in *Good Medical Practice* (GMC, 1995; RCGP, 1999) is the key. The new NHS health plan reflects this though it is still not clear how the development of effective appraisal throughout primary care is going to be developed and resourced.

Lastly, we look at clinical governance in its various guises and in particular the way in which general practice has dealt with poor performance, not just with practitioners but more widely with staff and fellow professionals.

Audit

The use and development of audit in general practice goes back many years but unfortunately, in spite of the millions of pounds invested, the next stage – and arguably the most important one of changing behaviour as a result – is often poorly developed. As we have seen in Chapter 4, practice decision making can be poor because of the inadequacy of the data available about process and outcomes. The use of national guidelines has been patchy, particularly in developing the role of the practice nurse. This often impinges on the practice's capacity to handle time and resource problems. The impact of the National Institute of Clinical Excellence (NICE) on the implementation and pursuance of guidelines could be significant in this area.

The simplest starting point is auditing what you do. It offers a chance to alleviate or remove those areas of everyday practice that cause frustration by identifying the facts surrounding them and using those facts to arrive at a clear solution, in order to change things. Taking time to find out the facts can, in the end, save time.

It is often seen as threatening and burdensome, threatening because people feel it will reveal things they would rather others did not know. Also being a somewhat blunt tool, it might only deal with those elements of the task that are measurable and ignore the essential 'soul' that may make up a considerable part of the service. It is vital to choose the subject for audit very carefully and make sure it is of relevance to all involved in order to get the facts and use them to create change.

Sometimes audits can be triggered by a significant event or by a patient complaint, or come from one particular interest of a partner, as shown in Example 39.

Example 39

A practice had started up a clinic to identify and monitor patients with hypertension. The partner running it was pleased with the results, but when challenged, defined that success in terms of the fewer patients he was seeing who needed only a blood pressure check. It became obvious that the degree of achievement of the real issue for the practice – namely getting patients with hypertension under control at appropriate levels – remained unclear. The other partners decided to carry out an audit of both the clinic and surgery interactions to test the success of the new system.

Box 6.1 summarises the common criteria for choosing an audit.

The art of audit is to match clarity about the way in which data can be collected and analysed with clarity of purpose. A practice has almost unlimited access to unlimited data, thanks to the computer. It is important not to waste time and resources

Box 6.1: Criteria for choosing an audit

- The problem is a common one.
- It affects patient care.
- It has consequences in terms of mortality or morbidity.
- Correcting the problem will save more money than ignoring it.
- The team has the skills and motivations to perform the audit.
- It is relevant to professional practice and development.

collecting data for the wrong, or no, purpose. Equally, it is important to remember that the source of data is only as good as the systems in place to ensure accuracy.

The use of audit to form the basis for decision making (*see* Chapter 4), to deal with performance issues, and to set standards and deal with complaints is not limited to clinical matters. For many of the areas that cause difficulties for general practice the need for good data lies in non-clinical areas, such as patient access. Indeed, the argument that runs through this book is that you cannot separate clinical and non-clinical anymore — if you ever could. This thesis makes it clear that audit should cover all aspects of an identified issue.

The sources of data include, of course, the medical record. It is easy and cheap to get access to data from this source in these days of computerised records, although there is also danger in relation to the analysis of those records. It is possible to alter notes and X-rays relatively easily to prove a point. In addition, data can come from sources such as the appointment register and hospital referral letters which are still in paper form. In looking at issues around doctor time it is invaluable to use simple data from past years, as shown in Example 40.

Example 40

The Middleton Surgery was worried about the delays in patient access to any doctor, let alone the doctor of the patient's choice. The average delay was two weeks, which they agreed was unacceptable. They had tried every combination of open and appointment-only surgeries, having longer 'extra' lists, a single doctor doing an open surgery, nurse telephone triage. The latter had simply tended to provide the patients with a new way round the receptionists.

The five partners took a whole day off a week and had eight weeks' holiday a year, including study leave. One partner had a half-time clinical appointment and one held only a three-quarter-time contract. When more partner time was suggested the partners merely said that patients would fill up any amount of appointments offered. It was also suggested that for a list of 10 000 they were not offering sufficient appointments, but this too was denied.

Eventually, the practice manager, after talking to a colleague from another practice, carried out an audit of the estimated number of appointments needing to be offered to meet the demand of the patients attending on the national average, tempered by the experience of the previous two years' figures. She worked on the following assumptions of acceptable standards for that particular practice:

● patients would be seen at five-minute intervals
● patient access should be at the standard of any doctor within
    48 hours, and the doctor of choice within seven days.

This gave the number of appointments needed. She then calculated the number of five-minute appointments that could be offered in the surgeries run within the doctors' current patterns of working. The doctors made it clear that they were not prepared to work on five-minute appointments but that they preferred to offer six consultations an hour. The practice manager recalculated on that basis. The shortfall was even greater. It was clear that they were short of doctor time to the tune of between eight and 11 sessions per week.

The partners were horrified and insisted that they could not achieve that without a reduction in income either by introducing more doctor time – another partner or assistant – or reorganising care to delegate further to other professionals. It was a vicious circle, but at least they had a clear idea of the size of the problem and the parameters to which they could work. In addition, the audit gave them a means of titrating the various options against the three variables – income, patient demand and doctor availability.

A regular programme of audits – covering clinical issues such as the monitoring of patients with chronic conditions – is now a regular part of many practices' lives. As we said at the beginning, the problem is that if the answers provided by the audit are unpalatable, then the audit circle tends not to be completed – in other words no action is taken to change the factors involved and therefore no change in service or quality is achieved. Arguably such audits are not worth doing in the first place – they cost time and effort without benefit.

To try to avoid this, the following questions have been found useful:

- is the nature of the problem for which the audit is to be used clear and agreed?

- is there a clear statement of the aims of the audit?

- is a range of methods tested before choosing the one to be followed?

- who is the audit for?

- is there a clear timescale?

- are the possible outcomes anticipated with plans for handling them?

Quality assurance and risk assessment

The development of quality-based patient services has to be a planned one, tailored to the particular needs of the practice. But there are some common themes that underlie the approach. Much of what has been said already applies to the ways in which standards of care and service should be agreed and articulated in the practice. They should be shared and communicated, written and agreed. Moreover, they should be made prior to any measurement of performance and should be achievable.

Preferably they should take into account patient needs and views as expressed through patient groups or, more bluntly, through complaints. It can be seen, therefore, that providing a quality-based service is an umbrella for the continuous staff development identified in Chapter 5 with equal emphasis on specifity and performance measurement that underpins good appraisal as described below.

As Kotter (1990) says, '... the planning process establishes sensible quality targets, the organising process builds an organisation that can achieve those targets, and a control makes sure that quality lapses are spotted immediately and corrected. Managerial processes must be as close as possible to fail safe and risk free'.

The emphasis on quality now has a government dimension and some resource allocation, unlike in the past. One of the main components of quality is local delivery of high-quality health-care, through clinical governance underpinned by modernised professional self-regulation and extended lifelong learning. Life-long learning is an investment in quality.

Example 41 shows what can be done.

Example 41

The McTeare Medical Centre had been in the forefront of developing audit locally and had a firm database for most of its activities. The team members were also keen to develop their interest in quality improvement. They recognised the need to complete the audit cycle to check that performance had improved. But they rarely had the time or energy to check that performance had improved, as the doing of the audits themselves took all their time.

They decided that they had to take stock. That stocktaking revealed that they were so busy starting new projects that they never completed any. They decided to draw up a quality improvement plan and asked one of the senior receptionists, who was a key player in the audit activity, to act as project co-ordinator. The practice manager was designated quality co-ordinator, and between them they were given the authority to devise the plan and, when agreed by everyone, to ensure that it was fully implemented and followed through. They were both sent on appropriate training courses and as a result identified the training needs of others. Between them they managed to change the culture to one of quality, rather than one of audit.

Accountability will not achieve quality improvement on its own. In a service with such a strong history of professional independence, collaboration has to be nurtured and supported through the approach of many different stakeholders, rather than being a simple matter of national prescription. Moreover, quality is a complex concept and different aspects of quality might have to be traded off against one another. Awareness of the different angles that different stakeholders have in relation to what is quality was well expressed by Øvretveit (1992), when he referred to the 'complex customer'. The importance given to new drugs by patients suffering from a condition which the drugs might alleviate will be different from the government looking at value for money across a range of conditions and treatments. Evaluation of the quality of treatment for the common cold will be different for doctors and patients. Government attitudes to the development of expensive but leading-edge, top-quality surgery for a rare condition will differ from that of the medical team developing it. Quality can be in the eye of the beholder and therefore the importance given to technical or clinical quality in relation to other factors relating to service delivery will have to be decided on a local collaborative basis. Practices working closely within PCGs have more hope of cracking this than those who insist on staying at arms' length and denying their underlying problem.

The following questions may be helpful:

● has the practice identified what is important to it in terms of quality assurance?

- has this been tested against other stakeholders in the practice, such as patients, the PCG or health authority and other colleagues?

- have the right methods for improving quality been defined and examined?

- does everyone who should be involved understand what is expected of him or her?

- have the conflicting elements within the standards set been recognised?

- is there a clear lead and co-ordinator for quality development?

Appraisal and discipline: what is wrong, not who is wrong

The exercise of accountability is primarily an exercise in appraisal, which is perhaps why appraisal as a management development tool has had a slow ingress in general practice, indeed in medicine generally. This is due in large part to myths and fears that exist about the way it can be used. Will it be essentially educational or essentially for discipline? These different purposes can come together when there are sensitive and difficult areas of performance and behaviour towards others to be managed. Such issues might include poor inter-personal skills in a receptionist or an inability to delegate in a practice manager. Example 42 shows this.

Example 42

Jane was a young receptionist who handled most aspects of her job extremely well. She had a very good manner with patients, be it at the front desk or on the telephone. She rarely lost her cool and was well liked by staff. The only problem was her attitude to the partners. She never smiled at any of them and frequently appeared to ignore their requests, although in fact she did what was asked quickly and without murmur. They thought she was rude and one or two described her as offensive.

The first appraisal meeting she had with the practice manager was an opportunity for the latter to deal with what was an inexplicable problem. With gentle encouragement, Jane revealed that she was terrified of the doctors. She had had a very painful and upsetting experience with a childhood illness, requiring long stays in hospital and many visits to doctors for painful treatment. Her illness had been effectively dealt with and she was very appreciative of what doctors had done – indeed her wish to work in a practice was due to this feeling of gratitude. But she was totally in awe and fearful of the partners.

The practice manager helped her talk about it and to see how her response to the partners affected others. Jane agreed that the practice manager could talk to the doctors about the issue and in turn some of the GPs felt able to talk to Jane. All of them modified their attitude to her and she became less fearful and more open in dealing with them.

As a management tool it is 'a process of enhancing self-awareness and sensitivity to others by providing feedback on personal performance' (Haman and Irvine, 1997). Giving people the opportunity through skilful interviewing to discuss performance and development is one of the most effective means of motivating them (*see* Chapter 5). Moreover, it gives managers a formal opportunity to assess how individual members of staff can best contribute to achieving the objectives of the practice, to identify areas where there is a duplication of effort, to identify obsolete activity, to create new challenges and to agree any skill needs.

It is a combination of regular, but informal, assessments throughout the year as people go about their daily business, and may include a review of issues of discipline and poor performance dealt with during the year at the time of occurrence. The centrepiece of appraisal, however, is the formal, semi-structured discussion between the member of staff being appraised and their manager or managers. This needs to be prepared carefully on both sides so that the best is obtained from this precious protected time, with everybody being clear what the purpose is and the range of possible outcomes. It is a time for frankness, clarity and constructive praise. It is not a 'pass/fail' assessment or a collection of 'Brownie' points. Box 6.2 lists possible purposes of any appraisal scheme.

Box 6.2: Purposes of an appraisal scheme

- To identify good performance.
- To identify and correct factors impairing performance.
- To develop a more collaborative style of management.
- To review the structures in place.
- To identify potential.
- To identify training and development needs.
- To reinforce present behaviour.

There are mutual benefits to a well-run and well-regarded scheme – for the organisation and the individual. Clearly the practice would look for improved communication and relationships, particularly between the staff and the person or people doing the appraisal, and it can be a good way of ensuring that the views and ideas of the staff are brought to the fore. All these benefits are important elements in enhancing the way staff work across inter-professional boundaries, within and outside the practice (*see* Chapter 5), and thus develop the general efficiency and effectiveness of the practice through raised morale.

But for the individual the benefits can be even more extensive. Feedback is important for the effective performance of any individual, feedback on their own contribution and also the chance to give feedback on how it feels to be managed in that particular organisation. The appraiser not only appraises but is appraised. Example 43 gives one such instance.

Example 43

Mary, the office manager, was very uncertain in her new role. This uncertainty filtered through to the receptionists and administrative staff she supervised. She was tentative in her allocation of work and rotas, and not always clear in her delegation. The staff therefore felt tentative themselves and errors increased. When she appraised Thelma, one of the receptionists, she raised the question of number of errors Thelma had made. Thelma responded by saying she was never clear what Mary meant and anyway when she did give her a job, Mary then stood over her and made her nervous. They discussed several examples of this that had occurred in the previous weeks.

Mary felt the point that Thelma was making was justified and shared with Thelma some of her own unsureness in finding her way into her new role. She enlisted Thelma's help in building up the whole team's confidence and in supporting her. They also identified areas where Thelma genuinely had a training need and made arrangements to get that met quickly.

Box 6.3 lists some of the benefits to individuals that can arise from good appraisal.

Time is the biggest resource needed to design, train for and implement an effective appraisal system, and that is a commodity that is in short supply in practice. Similarly, time equals

Box 6.3: Some benefits of an appraisal scheme to the individual

- Providing insight into personal motivators.
- Clarifying expectations.
- Improving effectiveness.
- Clarifying roles and boundaries between individual responsibilities.
- Reinforcing views of the organisation's fairness and consistency.
- Presenting opportunities to consider and formulate developmental plans.
- Allowing self-appraisal.
- Producing action plans.
- Helping to identify and manage stress.

money – training is the most overt and easily calculated expense. But the benefits of the investment needed are incalculable. If done properly, performance appraisal is a valuable management tool for improving the individual and therefore the practice. Schemes which are not designed well, not tailored for the particular practice needs, not introduced sensitively, do not have trained exponents and the outcomes of which are not followed through are certainly not worth the investment, and can be disastrous for both appraiser and appraisee.

Similarly, the other tool of accountability, that of discipline, is often exercised poorly. Handling the minority of cases of poor behaviour or performance is equally important and sensitive, and requires equally robust and well thought out procedures and training.

It is important to see disciplinary procedures, certainly in the initial stages, as another method of improving performance, not as a means of punishment. The purpose should be as much to encourage others to improve and hopefully rehabilitate the offender as to rectify faults and punish. It is to give a vital message to others that inadequate work will not be tolerated and to ensure that motivated and conscientious employees do not become disillusioned by seeing others 'get away with it'.

The impact of not being prepared to deal with poor performance or behaviour is therefore considerable. Not only does it impact on others in the organisation, but it can also have disastrous effects on the practice's relationship with the outside world and its standing in a community. This usually occurs when a practice has failed to grasp the nettle early enough and finds itself taking hasty decisions leading to litigation and tribunals. The unwillingness of GPs to face potential conflict and, on occasions, be intentionally tough and confrontational has been the downfall of many practices, as explored in Chapter 3. The downfall may result at worst in a finding against them at an employment tribunal or compensation in court, through to a loss of community standing, the retention of a poorly performing member of staff and disgruntled other staff with low morale.

The law and practical advice on the detail of the disciplinary framework desirable in a practice and the effective management of under-performing staff can be found elsewhere (Haman and Irvine, 2000). In general, the effect on accountability can be countered by having an agreed and published performance, disciplinary and grievance procedure, so that all in the practice know what is likely to happen in specified circumstances. It is far better for staff relations if disciplinary rules and procedures are established before rather than after an event. Apart from the view a tribunal might take of an employer without such rules, in terms of management practice, it is important that everyone knows the rules relating to work and the penalties for breaching them.

This discussion has been entirely about staff appraisal and discipline as it is rare for any practice to have a system of peer appraisal. There are schemes afoot to help partnerships develop such systems (Jelley, 1999), but they are very limited and may be overtaken, if not distorted, by the form of appraisal being introduced by the government. They relate more to the ability of partners to confront each other behaviourally than to the sort of formal process needed for employees. Similarly, the issue of discipline for partners is largely dealt with through the partnership contract. 'Whistle blowing' on partners, even where health is the issue, is also rare and similarly inhibited by the unwillingness to confront and handle conflict. Clinical governance will make a difference, but in our experience it has always been possible to use existing mechanisms for professional regulation to deal with a poorly performing partner *if* the partnership so wished. Without the right kind of culture, it is not clear that clinical governance will make much difference.

The whole art of dealing with accountability appropriately, be it through appraisal or discipline, is to be open, fair, consistent and prepared. Confidence in both appraisal and discipline requires effective operators, people trained and confident in what they are doing. The issues set out above around appraisal and discipline affect the underlying problem of identifying and enforcing accountability within general practice as a single organisation. It is interesting to relate them to the underlying issue of accountability of the practice and the doctors in it to the outside world. The issue of clinical governance is briefly highlighted below.

But first, here are some check questions to enable a practice to begin the process of reviewing this aspect of accountability.

- Does your practice have a formal appraisal system for the staff?

- Was it designed and agreed by the whole practice?

- Is it implemented regularly to an agreed timescale?

- Have the appraisers been formally trained?

- Is there regular follow-up (e.g. training development planning) as a result of appraisals?

- Is the system regularly reviewed and amended in the light of experience?

- Do the partners have a scheme for appraising themselves?

- Are there agreed and published disciplinary and grievance procedures?

- Have they ever been used and reviewed as a result of use?

The impact of clinical governance

Clinical governance as a concept is one of the national developments that is likely to have passed by most practices, except those already involved with the PCG. Its impact, however, is likely to be great and Chapter 11 speculates further on that. Its relevance here lies in the fact that it pulls together many of the strands of accountability in so far as they affect the NHS framework and reinforces a lot of the work that has already gone on in general practice over the years. It is a framework 'through which NHS organisations are accountable for continuously improving the quality of their services and safeguarding high standards of care, by creating an environment in which excellence in clinical care will flourish' (Roland and Baker, 1999). Clinical governance is about every member of staff recognising their role in providing high-quality care, using the most suitable method of providing that care, identifying every aspect of that care that needs improvement, making plans to improve it and monitoring success in so doing.

In other words, clinical governance is about being accountable to a force outside the practice for the care delivered within that practice. The importance of the subject for this chapter lies in the fact that if the quality of audit, quality assurance and internal performance review are well-developed, then clinical governance is merely a validation of that quality. However, if accountability is not recognised as an underlying issue within a practice, then it is clinical governance that will discover it. Clinical governance is about managing a practice well to provide high-quality care. Case Study C in Chapter 9 illustrates the impact of clinical governance, as does Example 44 below.

Example 44

Prentice Health Authority in developing its HImP had selected coronary heart disease as a priority. It asked all the PCGs to look at the guidelines in line with the NSF. When the PCG approached the Glendyr Practice, the partners were anxious about what would be expected of them, as they had not done many audits before. They were also rather resentful as they objected to the health authority dictating what they should and should not concentrate on. However, the health authority persuaded the partners that it was required of them now and arguing was a waste of time.

The partners were still clear that they would not do anything themselves but saw it as a purely administrative exercise, a bit like the old targets exercises, they thought. They told their practice manager to go to a local seminar on clinical governance and find out what was involved. She came back enthused and knowledgeable, and offered to be the clinical governance lead in the practice. The partners willingly – and in ignorance – agreed. She was given responsibility by them to draft plans for implementing the guidelines. She set to with a will and talked to the practice nurses to find out what problems they thought it would cause. A lot of the guidelines were new and unfamiliar, so she suggested that one of the local cardiologists come to talk to the nurses and doctors. She sold it to the doctors by saying that she could get PGEA approval for the hour, and that the nurses would be able to record the time for their PREP profiles. The talk was very successful and the partners began to be involved and interested, against their inclinations. They had a meeting with the practice manager and the nurses to discuss improving performance in this area. They were now seeing the exercise as something that was good for their patients not simply an exercise.

They decided that they had to get information on patients with angina, and set themselves the target of increasing to 95% the proportion of patients with angina who were known to be taking aspirin regularly. They also decided that they must increase to 90% the proportion of patients with hypertension whose blood pressure was controlled within prescribed limits.

They monitored their performance monthly and began to identify where and with whom there were problems. One partner's performance was below average and she agreed to attend some PGEA sessions on hypertension with one of the nurses. One of the receptionists who helped the nurses obtain the monitoring data had an appraisal interview in which she declared herself willing to enhance her computing skills. As a result she was able to take much workload off the nurses.

Clinical governance underlines many of the issues we have discussed in the four areas of underlying concerns that have arisen over the 18 years we have been carrying out diagnostic consultancy. It could be seen to provide a 'top-down' framework for accountable action alongside the 'bottom-up' development of environments for clinical excellence (Dewar, 2000). It covers themes around consistency, accountability, quality improvement and assurance, appraisal and management of poor performance, and working across boundaries both professional and public. Indeed inter-professional collaboration is central to achieving clinical governance. The activities involved are wide-ranging and cover all aspects of the practice. There is no need, however, to tackle them all at once, and although some priorities may be set externally, the practice still has to sort out its own priorities for improvement and development within that. A planned, staged approach will be best.

Box 6.4 sets out some of the components of clinical governance.

Box 6.4: Some components of clinical governance

- Clinical and organisational audit.
- Significant event auditing.
- Information systems.
- Risk management.
- Patient complaints.
- Professional development needs and training.
- Planning and prioritising.
- Handling poor performance.

The art is not to be overwhelmed by the range. Many of the components are covered by the underlying issues set out in these chapters. These are issues that practices have been tackling over many years – they are not new. What is new is that accountability for their delivery is now specifically external and to the state, as well as internal and to the individual practice organisation.

Frequent recommendations arising out of the underlying issue of accountability

Following from the above discussion of the underlying issues around accountability, the most frequent suggestions for improving this aspect of care have been as follows:

- develop a quality improvement plan within which a regular, prioritised audit cycle is developed, with clear standards for performance

- identify a responsible person in the practice to move the plan and its components forward, someone who will be able to take the clinical governance agenda forward

- design and implement a staff appraisal scheme and train appraisers appropriately

- ensure all good employer policies, including discipline and grievance, whistle blowing and complaints procedures, are in place and reviewed regularly

- take some collective responsibility for the performance of individuals, be they partners or staff, as well as for the performance of the team as a whole.

Part 3
Case studies

Introduction

Chapters 3–6 described the major management problems that the practices we have visited have faced and are still facing. The following four chapters contain four case studies that illustrate what has been described.

The case studies are pictures of real practices, suitably anonymised to protect those individuals who over the years have let us see how they work without let, hindrance or restriction. But the problems, issues and resolutions that they describe are real and many readers will recognise them. We have included these case studies because our experience of using the case study approach as the basis for role-playing and for other teaching materials is that the extended examples ring uncannily true to a wide range of doctors and staff.

The starting point in Case Study A (Chapter 7) is a diagnostic visit that revealed underlying issues about structures. Case Study B (Chapter 8) illustrates a practice with planning needs met by pursuing a practice and personal development programme. Case Study C (Chapter 9) is another example in which diagnostic consultants were called in for a full review and report, which reflected some of the underlying issues described in Part 2, particularly in relation to developing a common philosophy and set of values. The final case study in Chapter 10 illustrates the value of, and processes involved in, experiencing protected time away from the daily grind of practice, a recommendation that has resulted from more diagnostic visits than any other experiences.

References are made where appropriate to the text covering the issue illustrated, as indeed readers were referenced to a particular case study when reading the earlier part of the book. At the beginning of each case study the key areas illustrated are flagged for ease of reference. They form a bridge between the previous diagnostic and analytical part of the book and Part 4, which looks to the future and reflects how the lessons of the past have relevance for that future.

7
Case Study A
Rhondda Medical Group

Points illustrated

- How to identify and create effective management structures
- The importance of coherent teamworking through managing and communicating across professional groupings
- How to achieve explicit standards and accountability – governance

Description

Rhondda Medical Group is a four-doctor partnership working in a large industrial town, serving a population of 7000 people, mainly employed by three large factories on the outskirts of the town. The partners form a strong, cohesive group and obviously like and respect each other. They are all generally open-minded and seem willing to both listen and learn. They are keen to challenge each other freely and courageously, and their instincts are to be fair and objective. The senior partner was the leader and instigator of change. He was the trainer in the practice and vice chair of the LHC.

The nursing team provide a wide range of services in a cohesive team. The partners place a lot of confidence in the team, which means that the nurses tend to operate independently of the rest of the practice and run their own appointments system.

The receptionists form a strongly cohesive group and support each other. Rather than have specific rotas and duties allocated in advance, they work on a system of discussing with each other their availability on a week-by-week basis. They all keep an eye on what needs to be done, be it dealing with patients coming for appointments, telephone queries, getting out notes, repeat prescriptions and so on, and fill in where there is a gap. Reception tends, therefore, to look chaotic but they all use their initiative and take pride in the fact that everything is cleared every day. Patients' files are always up to date, telephones are answered within four rings, and patients are dealt with quickly and firmly, if not always with total patience. The doctors and patients do not complain.

The practice manager was appointed three years ago. She is a financial wizard, coming from a banking background, but she has found the clinical and people management side of practice management very hard. She has a deputy practice manager who deals with most of the staff issues and acts as senior receptionist. The partners are very happy with the level of drawings the practice manager achieves for them and the practice accountant has nothing but praise for her.

The premises are old-fashioned but an extension built recently has helped to give better treatment room facilities. The extension is reached by a glass-covered walk-way, so the nurses can be very isolated. The practice manager's office is also in the new extension.

The partners are keen to develop their management skills and recognise that the partnership currently has little team structure. Decisions are theoretically by consensus and dissension rarely causes a problem for the partners, who tend to avoid disharmony by deciding on the lowest common denominator. There is no real scheme of delegation to individual partners, although the senior partner keeps an eye on the finances and the junior female partner is the designated staff partner.

Presenting issues

The partners feel that the practice manager has lost her motivation. There are increasing staff complaints about minor and major matters, ranging from the temperature in the staff room to rates of pay. Also, the partners feel that there is a level of disharmony within the practice and are anxious that their own lack of management skills is contributing to this. They have asked external consultants to look at this.

Process

The consultants started their visit by having a tour of the building with the practice manager, admiring the new extension, and absorbing the atmosphere and the way the different teams reacted to her. She was fairly uncommunicative and was pleased to hand them over for the first formal interview with the senior partner. They interviewed all the partners individually before they returned to interview the practice manager.

The partners' perceptions of the issues facing the practice were clear from the interviews. Questions to them focused on:

- each partner's perceptions of the strengths and weaknesses of the practice
- what contributed to both
- what changes they would like to see and why.

The consultants made it clear to the partners that they could not assess an individual's performance and were not there to make judgements about the fitness of individuals for their posts.

As these interviews progressed they gained a lot of information about the practice and in particular how the partners saw their management responsibilities and the work of the practice manager. The interview with the practice manager was difficult as she was very reticent and unforthcoming. She clearly felt threatened and anxious and, in spite of the reassurance the consultants gave, did not feel able to open up. She saw her job as being primarily to keep the practice income up. She took pride in the fact that accounts were submitted on time and the partners' drawing was sustained. She was resistant to spending money on equipment and additional staff.

The interviews with receptionists and nurses were very open and informative, once the rules of confidentiality were established and the point was made firmly that the purpose of the visit was not to assess and pass judgement on the performance of individuals. It was clear that everyone was very concerned about the state of morale in the practice, and most of the staff ascribed this to the failure, as they saw it, of the practice manager to pull the individual teams together.

Without exception, all reception staff and most of the nurses quoted three issues as examples of poor management and communication, leading directly to the loss of morale and poor atmosphere. They were:

- the cancellation by the partners at the last minute of the practice Christmas dinner, said to be because of a lack of interest

- the change in staff uniform, allegedly without consultation

- the imposition of a Saturday morning rota for reception and nursing staff, again allegedly without consultation.

In spite of this coherence in identifying common grievances, each staff grouping, be it partners, nurses or receptionists, all resented the behaviours of the other teams.

The nurses felt that the reception team ran the practice for their convenience and did not help the hard-pressed nurses. They thought the doctors were largely competent, but felt that their (the nurses') worth was not recognised, nor was there any appreciation of how overworked they were.

The receptionists thought the doctors were only interested in having time off and getting in and out of the practice as quickly as possible, leaving the receptionists to deal with difficult patients. They felt undervalued and poorly paid, considering the contribution they felt they made to the practice income.

The partners in turn felt excluded from the reception area by the strong 'them and us' attitude of the receptionists. They resented the fact that if they wanted anything changed it met with resistance from the receptionists. They were puzzled that, in spite of the latitude they gave nurses clinically, they still seemed to complain about the workload and the support they got.

All three groups tended to exclude the practice manager from their particular team and saw her as a hindrance rather than a support. The receptionists felt that they did not need her. They were unable to describe any standards to which they all adhered, nor could they make any concerted or reliable comment about the workload, either of the practice as a whole or individual partners. They felt that trying to develop or follow common, clear policies and keep data on the key issues would lead to a worsening of relations between partners. It would reveal how each partner compared with the others. The receptionists were also clear that the practice was only small, so it was not necessary to set up a whole auditing paraphernalia, and anyway the partners would not invest any money whatever the results.

The nurses were more protocol-minded, but they followed the protocols learned on courses and these were rarely discussed with the GPs. They accepted that there was little clinical discussion in the practice and that their independence meant that the partners did not really know what they did and to what standard they worked. They felt that more explicit statements about standards of care and workload and performance would add to the enjoyment and their own sense of value, but they feared the process.

The partners were all very keen on audit and several had carried out their own small audits on specific disease management. Whenever they had suggested a joint nurse and partner clinical meeting, the nurses stated that they had no time. The partners were afraid of upsetting the receptionists because they were such a coherent team, operating it appeared very efficiently. They were afraid to disturb their routines in case they all fell apart. They recognised the issues that were being raised by clinical governance and the need for explicit standards and shared data on performance both as a practice and individually.

They delegated the running of the practice to the practice manager and were clear that she was responsible for setting the employment culture, in so far as they recognised one. They were unhappy that she appeared to be less effective in this aspect of her job but did not see what they could or should do.

The practice manager had read a lot about clinical governance and because of her business background was quite excited by it. She felt, however, that she would never persuade the component parts of the practice to adopt a single, coherent approach. She was unsure how the partners saw her role in managing the reception and even the nursing team, and did not feel accountable for the work of anyone else in the practice, beyond the deputy practice manager and the accounts clerk. The deputy practice manager was responsible for the personnel issues in the practice and the practice manager felt that it was the deputy, therefore, who set the employment culture in the practice. She did not, however, see that her responsibility for her deputy included the performance of the reception staff or the overall management performance standards in the practice.

In the course of the interview with the consultants she began to look at this issue afresh and became anxious about the implications for the way she and the practice might have to change.

Diagnosis of underlying issues

The partnership

1 The first underlying issue for the practice derives from the nature of the partnership and the relations between the partners and others. The partners resist accepting that they are the management board of the business, the employers, the owners and the people who make the final decisions and are held at law accountable for them, whether they make them directly or indirectly through others. Effective delegation therefore has to be differentiated from dumping or abdicating.

2 The partners are very open about their own lack of confidence in managing the practice. Unfortunately, this very openness has given rise to a fundamental lack of confidence in management within the whole practice. Anyone trying to exercise management skills across the whole practice meets resistance or positive hostility borne of fear of disrupting the effectiveness each professional team has developed for themselves within their own safe area of operation.

3 The partners have no formal team structure within the partnership to model for the rest of the practice or to demonstrate their responsibility for the overall activity and performance within the practice. The senior partner takes a lead with the practice manager on the finances of the practice, and the newest female partner, in desperation, has taken on the role of staff partner. But these are not recognised formally and no partner takes a lead on nursing or receptionist development in the practice, or for developing the practice's

response to clinical governance issues. The trainer among the partners has not had a registrar for two years so there are no new ideas coming in to help the partners review how they work.

4 Consequently, there is little effective management of the practice manager. She is not clearly managed by one partner, not even the most senior. Indeed, she can find herself responding to four different requests and agendas. She does not feel empowered to manage up to the partnership or to model good management practice.

5 The partners have limited success in confronting difficult issues. They have a natural reluctance to be tough on people with whom they work closely, and can give mixed and fudged messages to the staff as a consequence. Their own lack of knowledge of the legal and good practice boundaries around employment issues further undermines the partners' confidence in their own management abilities and means they neither see nor understand the implications of some of the existing poor employment practice. They seem not to expect, demand or get timely advice from the practice manager on these issues and, not surprisingly, she therefore believes herself absolved of responsibility for them. The issues of uniforms, Christmas parties and Saturday working are prime examples here. All three issues went wrong because of inexperience and lack of management confidence and knowledge of employment law and practice, as well as the lack of clear personnel procedures within the practice.

6 The partners believe that they delegate effectively and that by leaving people to get on they are demonstrating trust and confidence. In fact, delegation quickly becomes dumping or abdication of responsibility if it is not accompanied by empowerment to change, authority and resources (see Chapter 4). The nurses can provide more services if they are

not so overloaded and the receptionists can deliver the standard of patient access the partners want, but the partners have to be specific about their aims and monitor what happens. Similarly, delegation within the partnership is lacking formality and authority to act and decide within prescribed, described and communicated limits on behalf of the whole partnership.

The practice management team

1 It is not clearly understood that the management of the practice is the responsibility of all who operate on behalf of the partnership in any way. The focal points are of course those who set the framework of policy, usually the partners, and the practice manager, who is responsible for ensuring that that policy is translated into service on a day-to-day basis.

2 There is a lack of an explicit job description for the practice manager, who consequently could not be clear what was expected of her by the partnership as a whole and how she was to be managed herself.

3 The practice manager manages the reception and administrative staff through the deputy practice manager. Because the practice manager has no job description there is no clear job description for this post either, with all the attendent woolliness.

4 If there are expectations of the practice manager that are outside her current expertise and experience there is no plan currently to provide her with the skills and knowledge needed.

5 The senior nurse has no direct line to the partnership as a whole, but tends to catch whichever partner is around when a problem arises. The management of the nursing team is left to the nurses themselves, which leads to confusion of

treatment between the nurses and individual partners, and confusion over the manning of clinics. This is another aspect of delegation becoming dangerously close to abdication.

Practice culture

1   Underlying all issues is a strong 'them and us' culture. The partnership is a very strongly bonded group of like-minded people who enjoy working together. This is a great strength but, as with the reception team, it can lead to vast gulfs between different specialisms within what is effectively one team.

2   All this tends to lead to exclusivity and resentment, as well as poor communication. There are individual agendas rather than everyone working in one team to the same end. The practice manager has no team to join and her deputy tends to belong to the staff team, thus isolating the practice manager even more.

3   In addition, there is a cohort of long-serving staff with strong personalities and personal ownership of the practice. They appear to be somewhat disaffected and to resent any attempt to manage them. They seem to use requests for change or change itself as opportunities to exercise their power over the practice, the partners, the practice manager and her deputy, and in some instances their colleagues.

Discussion and recommendations

The practice has enormous strengths to build on and a strong base from which to develop the areas cited above. The partners had spent time out of the practice together before and it was now time to create another opportunity to consider the whole of the diagnostic consultancy experience in a protected environment. The interviews, the feedback session and the written report had begun the process of enhancing the partners' management skills, particularly in the area of managing people. A list of the basic areas covered in terms of management (Appendix 3) was given to the partnership to form the basis for part of their discussions.

It is essential to begin the process of empathising and sharing across the artificial boundaries that have been created. They need to work through the components of the management of the practice (from policy decisions around employment policies to the colour of the examination couch curtains) and look at the potential for delegating as far as possible to the people actually carrying out the tasks.

The practice needs to ensure that it is equipped in personnel skills and has confidence in the legal framework and best practice within which it operates as an employer. Furthermore, the management team should feel emboldened to share their initial thoughts with the rest of the staff through a practice development process, which could involve everyone in devising and owning the future (*see* Case Study B in Chapter 8). The issues that would be included in such a programme would be:

- the development of a fully worked through and discussed appraisal system

- the provision of training interviews and training plans for all members of staff

- the organisation of regular opportunities for people to exchange knowledge and skills with other members of the practice to ensure empathy and understanding between them all

- ways of establishing the confidence of all that constructive criticism and confronting will be supported and followed through.

The practice shows itself, in principle, to be very committed to quality service. In order to ensure that its understanding of clinical governance and quality is coherent and uniform, specific training and development is needed. Many of the areas that need to be enhanced are already being developed in the practice, such as audit, appraisal, and training and development. However, they need to be brought together in a coherent way that makes clear the authority and responsibilities delegated with that responsibility.

The team needs to review its approach to risk management and auditing significant events that have occurred, and find ways of introducing patients' views into these discussions.

Recommendations

1   The partners should arrange another time out of the practice to stand back from the pressures of everyday practice and review the findings of the consultants' report.

2   That occasion should be used to identify and describe the management team and its responsibilities, dealing with the following issues:

- the setting of targets for the next three years
- the sort of management needed to achieve them
- how much the partners want to do themselves as a group
- how much to delegate and to whom
- the job descriptions that go with such delegation both within the partnership and to those outside it
- the skills needed by the delegatees
- the skills available in the practice
- how to fill the gaps between the latter two.

3   Regular team meetings for representatives of all parts of the practice as well as management team meetings are needed, initially on a weekly basis, to discuss current live issues.

4 They need to agree standards of performance through clear and written targets to prevent misunderstanding and monitor performance against them effectively, and to share these with the staff.

5 The practice manager and the partner designated responsible for personnel issues, together with other staff in managerial and supervisory positions, need to improve their personnel skills and knowledge through work-based case study discussion and analysis in protected and expertly facilitated time.

6 The current staff handbook, contracts of employment and disciplinary procedures should be sent to the personnel consultant for an up-to-date view on their accuracy, robustness and flexibility.

7 The practice should work towards holding a practice development programme that would include all members of the team and enable them to fit their personal development into and around the agreed priorities of the practice.

8 It is suggested that the practice manager be given the task of joining the LHC Quality and Clinical Governance Team and at the weekly practice meetings have a protected slot to share her learning and discuss areas for development.

Short-term outcomes

The partners arranged to have a weekend (Friday evening to Saturday evening) with skilled facilitators to work through their problems – how they managed themselves and the practice manager. As a result, they set up a loose structure within the partnership, designating one partner as the managing partner, whose responsibility it was to manage the practice manager and be her first point of reference. The partners committed themselves not to interfere in this relationship and to give permission to each other to challenge any behaviour that undermined it. They selected the most junior female partner for this task.

They decided to allocate responsibility for managing the nursing team to a named partner, to whom the senior nurse would report. That partner was given responsibility with the nurses to develop nursing policy and practice and bring a report on that strategy to the partnership. They rejected the idea of a senior or lead partner, but the nominal senior partner would go on doing the finances.

They recognised that the practice manager had been left unsupported and that her job was inadequately defined. They agreed the outline of her responsibilities and delegated to the new managing partner responsibility for drawing up the detail with the practice manager. They decided to review the work-load of the staff — management, administration, reception and nursing. They set up a small working group of partners, practice manager, a receptionist and a nurse to do so, and asked a local practice manager to work with this team to write a report on both numbers and workload, and also on the implications for income and expenditure.

This was also a first attempt to break down the culture of 'them and us' by getting people to work together. They reported back to the practice manager and to an open staff meeting. The response was guarded but there was a recognition that they were at least trying to do something to organise themselves.

Longer-term outcomes

The arrangements worked well for a time, but the partners were unable to stick to their commitment not to interfere, and there were several heated exchanges between the managing partner and the others when they did so. However, this of itself meant that the partnership was beginning to handle confrontation. The working group was very successful and produced good ideas, which were workable and affordable. They were implemented, which gave the staff confidence and gave the partners a feeling of dealing with issues.

The practice manager and senior nurse both attended a seminar on appraisal schemes and the personnel consultant helped them devise and introduce an appraisal programme as part of an overall review of personnel policies. This took over a year with consultation and it included the regular appraisal of the practice manager by the managing partner. Training needs were identified from this process and she undertook further developmental courses. The managing partner herself identified her need for management training and became so interested she undertook the Diploma in Management Studies.

Overall, practice morale improved significantly as people began to work more across boundaries and the enhanced skills of those managing the teams improved the quality of life in the practice for those in the front line. Regular partnership away days were held each year and whole practice development opportunities were developed (*see* Case Study B).

8
Case Study B
Newtown Health Centre

Points illustrated

- How to develop a practice plan
- How to ensure personal development plans are created
- How to work across boundaries
- How to implement change

Description

The Newtown Health Centre comprises a three-doctor partnership in a commercial inner-city area with a high incidence of single-parent families, teenage pregnancies and smoking. There is also a large elderly population, with a lot of respiratory disease from the local steelworks.

All but Thursday morning surgeries are by appointment only, but with increasingly long lists of extras to cope with patient-defined emergencies. The premises are old and rather cramped, but provide a wide range of allied services, including well-woman and well-man clinics, an asthma clinic, and the services of a visiting geriatrician and dermatologist.

Two of the partners have worked together for ten years but the third partner is the last in a series of four different partners over the past five years.

The turnover of reception staff is also high, with only two of the six receptionists being at the practice for over three years. The practice manager is the senior partner's widowed sister and has been with her brother for nine years. The practice has an appraisal system and a regular practice meeting for all staff once a month, for which the practice closes for two hours.

Presenting issues

The practice decided to seek help in establishing a better team approach to its future planning as an organisation, through developing a practice plan and individual development plans for each member of the team. The partners are concerned at the turnover of both doctors and receptionists, and have noted that the nursing team of three have worked together for 13 years without a change. They want to find out how to replicate this across the practice and to improve their teamworking.

The health authority agreed to support the process as part of its plans to support CPD. It agreed with the practice's belief that such an exercise would bring together 'the different perception, information systems, contributions, skills and needs of the people who manage, deliver and receive health care in the community setting' (Elwyn and Smail, 1998). They recommended two facilitators to help with the process.

Process

The facilitators and the practice agreed that they should set success criteria for the project:

- that the practice should commit itself to the project by attendance on two away days and by carrying out homework undertaken between the two away days

- that each team member should emerge feeling that they had learnt something, changed in some way and valued participating in the project

- that the practice as a team would recommend the process to others.

The preparation

The facilitators visited the practice to meet the practice manager and discuss the arrangements for an introductory visit to the practice. The purpose of the visit was to identify the training and educational activities of individuals, and the changes and priorities currently and over the next five years.

Prior to the visit the facilitators asked for the following information:

- the practice leaflet and annual report

- management and organisational structure, either in narrative or diagrammatic form

- job descriptions for the practice manager, practice nurse, receptionist, secretary and, if available, health visitor and district nurse

- details of the partners and staff of the practice:
  - position
  - length of service
  - status, full-time/part-time
  - specialisms/outside activities

- any other relevant background information.

The purposes of the initial visit were:

● to introduce the consultants to the practice team

● to discuss the information that would be helpful for the first stage of assessing the current position of the practice and its individual team members

● to complete data questionnaires (Attachment 1) and interview, both individually and collectively, as many members of the practice as possible, in order to gain insight into the practice and its operation

● to collect any other information relevant to preparing for the first half-day away day.

The consultants conducted small group and individual interviews. In total, eight people were interviewed and the questionnaire was left for the four staff who were not available that day.

The first away day

The aims for the first away day were:

● to identify future needs, opportunities and potential development for the practice

● to enable individuals to identify personal, educational and developmental needs in that context.

Box 8.1 sets out the agenda for the afternoon and Box 8.2 contains the priorities and obstacles as gleaned from the preparatory work and which provided the basis of the afternoon.

The practice exhibited real teamwork in helping each other and worked through the issues to achieve the aims of the day. A number of priorities for the practice were agreed, to be worked up further before the next session. To facilitate this, the

Box 8.1

Newtown Medical Centre: Away day 1 – Programme

Aims: to identify future needs, opportunities and potential development for the practice, and enable individuals to identify personal, educational and developmental needs in that context.

13.00	Welcome and introductions	Plenary
	Ground rules and facilitators' role	
13.30	Practice aims and obstacles	Plenary
14.00	Overcoming the obstacles and achieving the aims	Small groups
15.00	Report back	Plenary
15.45	Tea	
16.00	Personal development needs	Trios
16.30	Next steps	Plenary
17.00	Close	

Box 8.2: Priorities and obstacles

Priorities for the practice:
- increase in health promotion and disease prevention
- gaining training practice status
- developing a nurse practitioner role
- a teamwork approach
- enhancing patient services, e.g. sports clinic, chemist on site.

Obstacles to progress:
- power devolving from general practice to PCG
- prescribing issues
- lack of audit
- poor computer system.

flip charts produced in small group and plenary sessions were photocopied later and circulated to each member. Homework, to be done before the second whole-day away day scheduled for a month later, was agreed and allocated.

The homework

The homework – working up the priorities with details of aims, targets, resources, timescales and named practice lead – was produced in good time and formed the basis of the agenda for the next away day. The consultants summarised the homework on overhead acetates and handouts. These acetates and the agenda for the day can be found as Attachment 2.

The second away day

The programme for the second away day is set out in Box 8.3.

Box 8.3

Newtown Health Centre: Away day 2 – Programme

Aim: to produce
● a practice development plan
● a personal development plan for each team member
● identify any further team development needs.

09.30	Coffee	
10.00	Introduction	
10.15	The five organisational developments and personal development plans	Plenary
10.45	Prioritising the practice plan	Small groups
11.15	Coffee	
11.30	Feedback and developing an action plan	Plenary
12.15	Lunch	
13.15	Personal development plans	Individual exercise
14.00	Small group discussion	
14.30	The review process	Plenary
15.00	Tea	
15.15	Evaluation exercise	Small groups
	Discussion	Plenary
16.30	Close	

The programme for the day was designed to:

- enable the practice team to prioritise their aims for the next three to five years
- identify the resources needed to achieve these aims
- identify individual and practice development needs.

As for the first away day, this day was structured to facilitate teamwork and to allow for the differing pace of work of the different team members. Individuals worked on their own, in small groups and in plenary sessions. The day was interspersed, as appropriate and when the opportunities presented themselves, with the facilitators reflecting on and initiating discussions on how the practice worked as a team.

The personal and practice development plans

The practice developed a comprehensive practice plan. It identified and agreed its priorities as follows:

- teamwork development
- health promotion, chronic disease management
- family planning
- becoming a training practice
- developing the nurse role to nurse practitioner status.

Each priority was worked through in small groups using flip charts and contained a list of activities needed to achieve the stated aim, a schedule of action with timescales and named persons who were responsible for either leading on the topic or helping the 'leader' achieve the aim/targets. The flip charts were later typed up by the facilitators to form the practice development plan.

In the last session, individuals were invited to complete a personal development plan using the form in Attachment 3. The participants were asked to consider their role in the achievement of components of the practice's overall plan and identify for themselves areas of training and development need. These first drafts were handed in to the practice manager for further discussion and to produce a practice training programme.

The quality of these plans was most impressive and of particular note was the commitment and imagination demonstrated by the practice receptionists. Their individual plans included such developments as helping team development by attending a course on communication skills, acquiring both knowledge and skill in audit, and participating in chronic disease management through learning more about that field from the partners.

Discussion and recommendations

Before the day ended, the participants were asked to reflect on their involvement in this project and to complete an evaluation form. A summary of this evaluation can be found in Attachment 4.

The practice and the consultants were satisfied that they had successfully achieved their objectives. Personal and practice development plans had been produced which were the result of real debate and discussion within the team, involving compromise and in some cases disappointment.

The practice worked with real commitment. The quality and timeliness of the homework was evidence of the practice team's hard work, commitment and understanding of the project.

The evaluation forms showed the participants' learning, the change they had undergone as a result of the project and the unanimous enthusiasm for recommending the process to others.

Short-term outcomes

The practice immediately diarised a monthly practice meeting to be held between 1.00 and 3.00 pm with a sandwich lunch provided. It was agreed that the agenda for the first hour would be formal, made up of issues put to the practice manager prior to the meeting. The second hour would be a training opportunity. To begin with it was agreed that each professional group in the practice would present their work and help the other practice colleagues understand what they did, how it interfaced with all other parts of the practice, and what could be done to help and support them. The health visitors offered to go first, followed the next month by the receptionists, and then the practice nurses. Eventually the partners were persuaded to give a session. These proved both popular and enjoyable, but also provided a stronger understanding and empathy between the groups. Problems of communication and misunderstanding were ironed out, and people felt able to challenge each other when attitudinal or behavioural issues got in the way of day-to-day working relationships.

In addition, the practice manger instituted a suggestion box scheme for patients and all members of the practice, which provided sensible and some frivolous ideas, many of which were followed through. For instance, the staff suggested that the practice manager maintain a master diary in her office of all activity in the practice, which anyone could access but not alter. A patient suggested how to increase privacy at the front desk through a simple resiting of a baffle board.

Longer-term outcomes

In the longer term, the practice manager drew up a regular training and development plan and the developmental aspirations of all members of the team were discussed at a practice meeting and tested against the practice priorities. For example, the partner who was interested in sports medicine deferred his course for two years, until other team members had done other more pressing training. He sought leave to attend the course, but did not expect the practice to meet the cost out of the training budget, as setting up a sports injury clinic remained a low priority for the practice.

A regular day out was taken by the practice to review the plans and priorities on a yearly basis.

The partners, therefore, were less beset by everyday problems of staff absence as the morale in the practice grew rapidly and staff turnover reduced. Their reputation as well-motivated, keen practitioners grew.

The practice manager started to enjoy the job and was able to put the practice forward for Investors in People successfully. She became chair of the local PCG Practice Managers' Forum and developed an interest in clinical governance.

For the staff, their personal development was enhanced as well as the skills and tools to do the jobs in the practice. They became well-motivated and brought a lot of initiative, and therefore challenge and change, to their jobs.

The other professionals similarly were better-motivated and the attached staff turnover reduced. Indeed, community staff vied to work for the practice and be so involved in its development.

For the health authority the practice became a frequently used organisation for pilots and experiments, and patient complaints were few and far between.

Attachment I: Practice and personal development plans. Individual data form

Name:

Job title:

Date of commencement:

Educational qualifications: Date

Professional qualifications: Date

Other training received:

Type of training   Subjects   Date
(on job, course, day release,
distance learning, etc.)

Other skills:

Membership of professional bodies:

For the partners

What do you see as the three main priorities for the practice over the next
five years?

What key developments must occur to achieve these priorities?

For the staff

What do you think are the main changes facing the practice over the next
few years?

What do you think has to happen in order to manage these changes effectively?

Attachment 2: Possible developments for next five years identified in homework

1   Training practice
Aim: to become a training practice.
Purpose: to bring new ideas and externally revalidate the practice.
Timescale: when a partner is eligible in four years' time.
Resources needed:
- library
- summarised and tagged records
- computerised system
- trainees!
- locums.
Costs: not worked out.

2   Family planning/counselling service
Aim: to avoid unplanned, unwanted pregnancies and subsequent health problems,
          e.g. depression.
Target population: women, especially teenagers.
Project:
- provide accessible clinics, including 'drop-in' service
- promote sexual health through education, screening and counselling
- offer range of contraception
- centralise monitoring of patients.
Resources needed:
- a third nurse
- a receptionist dedicated to the nursing team
- contraceptive devices – pills and IUCDs, etc.
Costs: not calculated.

3   Sports clinic
Aim: to set up a sports clinic to provide specialist service for those with
          sports injuries.
Target population: young males with sports injuries who currently go to A and E.
Resources and costs:
- skills training for doctor and nurse
- specialist equipment
- advertising
- extra receptionist time.
Costs: considerable!

4   Teamwork
Aim: to develop teamwork further.

Purpose: to increase the morale of all who work in practice, reduce the staff turnover, and increase co-operation and support over different working groups.
Means:
- continue developing protocol files
- monthly staff meetings
- bulletin board
- share knowledge of each other's and in-house providers' jobs
- patient suggestion box
- training through in-house, individual training plans, external training, nurse development training, professional development for doctors, e.g. MRCGP, GP refresher course, diploma in DT
- master diary kept in practice manager's office.

Resources: locums.
Costs: not worked out but would include exam and course fees.

5   Nurse practitioner
Aim: to extend the role of practice nurse to nurse practitioner.
Timescale: when one of the practice nurses is eligible (in three years).
Purpose:
- to release medical time
- to increase income-generating work
- to increase nurse participation in decision making and innovation in the practice
- to act as a resource for practice audit.

Means of working: through open surgeries and appointment system.
Resources needed:
- cover to allow practice nurse to qualify
- partner time to mentor
- a dedicated office/surgery
- a dedicated receptionist.

Costs: unknown.

6   Health promotion – chronic disease management
Aim: to reduce hospital admissions of asthma, diabetes and hypertensive patients by 50% by 2004.
Target population: at-risk patients, especially the young.
Project:
- establish a database to target patients at risk
- opportunistically through patient lifestyle questionnaires
- data from patients attending clinics and data from prescriptions
- offer health education at every opportunity
- conduct regular in-house audits to monitor progress.

Resources: health promotion equipment.
Costs: not calculated.

Attachment 3: Personal development plans

Name ....

Job Title ....

Subject/topic

Methods

By whom/organisation

Timescale

Success criteria

Attachment 4: Evaluation questionnaire

1   During this project (including today) what have you learnt about:

- yourself?
- your colleagues?
- working as a team?
- other organisations/people involved in the project?

2   What (if anything) has frustrated you about the project?
3   What have you most valued about participating in the project?
4   Would you recommend this process to others? Please give the reasons for your answer.

9
Case Study C
Ayrshire Road Health Centre

Points illustrated

- The importance of an explicit common philosophy and set of values (*see* Chapter 3)

- The need for leadership (*see* Chapter 3)

- Inappropriate behaviour and morale (*see* Chapter 3)

- Unstructured meetings and decision making (*see* Chapter 4)

- How the personality clashes between partners can disguise deeper underlying problems (*see* Chapter 4)

- How to address conflict appropriately and move forward (*see* Chapter 4)

- Delegation within the partnership (*see* Chapter 5)

Description

Ayrshire Road is a five-partner urban surgery with a relatively stable population, based on local low-tech industry and commerce. It is firmly rooted in the community, with good purpose-built premises and a long-standing partnership. The two most senior partners, Brian and Calum, have had significant major tensions between them over the past 10 years. These are perceived by the others as being due to the level of external activity of Brian and the perceived resulting workload of Calum, exacerbated by personality clashes between the partners themselves and their spouses. Consequently, there is a recognised vacuum in the leadership of the practice.

Despite this state of affairs, the practice is patient-oriented, with doctors very accessible to other members of the clinical practice team and to patients. They provide, together with the team of nurses, a wide range of clinical services. There is a welcoming and friendly atmosphere, largely because the staff group work as a team. They are led by a loyal and long-serving practice manager, Ella, who is nearing retirement. She has long given up trying to interfere with the 'ructions' in the doctors' room. The staff, receptionists, nurses and attached staff are frustrated and irritated by what they perceive as poor management by the partners. There is no consistency in the way the nurses are used by the partners or any common clinical protocols in use.

Partners allocate responsibilities among themselves, but the allocation lacks clarity, with different partners and staff having quite different perceptions of each partner's responsibilities. No one partner leads the team and no one partner regularly chairs meetings. It is a training practice and both senior partners are approved trainers. They rarely share the work of supervising the registrar, however, and as their mode of working is very different, the registrar received a very specific model from each. The other partners and practice manager also tend not to be involved much in the support of the registrar for fear of offending one of the two older partners.

It is a fundholding practice and has long practised 'benchmarking' itself through being a training practice; one of the partners obtained FbA of the RCGP, and another showed interest in the RCGP Quality Practice Award. Brian was largely responsible for fundholding, with a part-time fundholding manager who had since moved on to the PCG. Brian was very active in the development of the local PCT and had expected to be elected to it, even to be its chair. He was unsuccessful, largely because none of his partners supported him. As a result, his interest in that development had reduced and now the practice tended not to be involved with the PCT development.

Presenting issues

The poor management in the practice and their inability to deal with the partnership's dysfunction and lack of leadership frustrates the younger partners and the staff. There are murmurs of a partnership split and a haemorrhage of good staff. There is anxiety about what will happen when the practice manager retires. One of the older partners, Calum, sees the situation as untenable and wants help to resolve it (preferably by encouraging the other partners to dissolve the partnership and exclude Brian). Brian sees no point in reviewing what is going on in the practice as he does not intend to change, leave or retire. He sees himself as wronged, aggrieved and unvalued, and very sore at the lack of support for his election to the PCG, especially as he had worked so hard to make the practice successful at fundholding. He just wants to be left alone to do his clinical work.

Process

The consultants had an opening hour's discussion with Ella, the practice manager, to get an overview of the personnel and issues in the practice (see Appendix A for details of a diagnostic consultancy visit). In this discussion, Ella revealed that she would be retiring in the next few years. They also had a tour of the premises and a chance to meet the staff generally. They then worked through a timetable of interviews with all the partners individually and all members of the practice team who were available.

Confidentiality was stressed throughout the visit. It was made explicit to each interviewee that what was being said on both sides was confidential within the interview, unless explicit permission was given to convey it elsewhere. Care was taken to ensure that individuals' views were integrated and could not therefore be attributed to that one individual without consent.

The interviews took a similar shape with each interviewee, with some being more in-depth and longer than others, e.g. partners tended to take an hour, while the junior receptionist, who had only been at the practice for six months, took only 15 minutes. The shape of questions for the partners was as follows:

- why did the partners feel the need for external advice and support?

- what were the areas of strength and pride in the practice?

- what areas needed further development or change?

- what did the interviewee hope would happen as a result of the visit?

The non-partner interviews tended to concentrate on the first two points.

It was important to spend time at the beginning of the interviews putting interviewees at their ease and testing that they were genuinely describing their perceptions of the practice and not what they thought was suitable or expected of them. By and large all were very open and honest, and only the partners were tentative about what some saw as disloyal comments and thoughts they might have about colleagues. The interview process released inhibitions and gave them a chance to 'let off steam' and also to develop some thoughts about the way to move forward by establishing what lay behind the presenting issues.

The interviewers were able to build up a picture of the practice and test perceptions and views by getting corroboration or otherwise. Sensitive issues and common themes were drawn out and explored individually.

Diagnosis of underlying issues

1 There was considerable impact among staff and patients from the ongoing and very public personality conflicts between the two older partners, ranging from tolerant amusement to acute discomfort, diminishing the partnership and therefore the practice. Interviews revealed that these personality issues, and the way other partners dealt with them, were hiding deeper differences of values and philosophy within the partnership. These differences included:

- belief in the overriding importance of individual patient care as against a belief that population medicine is the primary concern of the practice team, for which the whole group has to take responsibility
- a doctor-centred, slightly old-fashioned approach, tending to encourage repeat consultations and personal patient lists as against a more team approach, delegating and sharing with the nursing and therapist professionals
- belief in providing full 24-hour care, based on minimal use of on-call rotas, as against using the opportunities provided by NHS Direct and walk-in clinics, as well as emergency doctor services, as ways of both improving patient access to care and providing partners with acceptable lifestyles
- a need to demonstrate, through validated quality assurance, that the practice is providing care of an acceptable standard as opposed to a belief that the time taken to collect data and analyse performance takes away doctor time from actually delivering the care
- a consistent and inclusive use of computers for data entry, retrieval and analysis, against an antipathy to the use of computers and data entry
- a belief in the use and development of performance appraisal and review to improve practice and personal performance, as opposed to resistance to more time spent

on examining performance and trying to measure it meaningfully when the major activity is seeing patients.

2 None of the partners was prepared either to exhibit leadership or accept the leadership of others. Brian and Calum, who had the skills and status to do so, were blocked by their personal rivalries; another partner lacked assertiveness skills and the other two doctors tended to push from behind rather than lead from the front.

3 Meetings, although frequent, were poorly chaired and tended to be sources of stress and conflict rather than debate and cohesion.

4 There was evidence of harassment of a partner by another and there were other examples of inappropriate conduct. People who had the power and position to confront destructive behaviours did not do so because of feelings of impotence, inappropriateness or fear of being attacked or snubbed.

5 The problems arising from the partner relationships and the leadership issues were further compounded by limited knowledge, skill and training in management. This gap was not recognised or acknowledged by all of the partners.

Discussion and recommendations

The interview process, by highlighting poor decisions or ineffective staff management, helped partners and the manager recognise where there are deficiencies in their management skills and experience.

This gap was exhibited in:

- the way meetings were conducted, as discussed above
- ineffective and sometimes inappropriate decision making where decisions were not always based on detailed knowledge of the subject

- unclear allocation of duties and responsibilities to each other
- lack of teamwork in the partnership itself and in the practice
- time management, where partners got involved in the comfort zone of operational management, such as data entry
- demotivating 'dumping' rather than delegation of tasks to all groups of staff.

The following recommendations were discussed and agreed as the first steps to moving forward.

1 The fundamental nature of the divisions revealed in the analysis meant that it was essential that the partnership reviewed openly and fearlessly the differences in the values and priorities of the partners, and established the baseline from which the way forward could be mapped.

 This could best be done in a safe environment away from the practice in protected time. This needed to be done through a facilitated day where time could be given to standing back from the practice, designed to enable the partnership to agree where the practice was going and to start to look at how to get there. This latter issue required commitments from each partner to change in some way.

2 The lack of leadership in the practice had led to:
- little strategic planning
- no sense of direction
- a sense of impotence and 'drift'.

Part of the time for thought being proposed was to include the way in which the equality between partners, held so dear by most of them, could be reconciled with the recognised and acknowledged implications of not having a leader as set out above. The planning and prioritising could be a corporate activity for the whole group, and the framework policies decided by them, but with effective delegation to one partner to represent the partnership to the staff and the outside world.

3   The allocation of responsibilities between the partners needed to be revisited and reviewed in the light of the decisions made at the time out. In particular, they needed to relate to the context of the major activities of the practice. They might be as follows:

- finance
- staff
- clinical development
- nursing policy
- external relations.

The allocation also needed to reflect the aptitudes and experiences of the partners, as well as predilection. The focus needed to be on providing the strategic direction of the staff, ensuring through effective delegation that doctor time and skill were used appropriately and prudently. Focus was to be on strategic direction for staff and not doing it themselves, but this greater clarity would enable rudimentary concepts of accountability and appropriate delegation to be applied (*see* Chapter 5).

4   Part of the time out recommended above was to address the system of chairing the different practice meetings and the chairing skills of the partners. This was used as a proxy to demonstrate the effectiveness of good leadership in the narrow setting of a discussion. Chairing is a highly skilled activity and one of the major elements of leadership in an operational organisation like a practice. Training in chairing skills was recommended for at least one of the partners.

5   There were many different types of practice meeting, all of which needed to be well-chaired to ensure the purpose was clear, everybody's feelings were respected and everyone felt they had had their say. For the regular clinical and

business meetings there needed to be a clear record of the decisions reached, and the implementation and achievement of such decisions monitored at subsequent meetings.

6   The issues of potential harassment of one partner by another, and the legal implications of the behaviour of Calum and Brian in inhibiting the work of others, needed to be talked through, particularly with the more junior partners, and the underlying fears and inhibitions articulated and explored. The three junior partners now needed to build on their confidence in identifying the presenting problems and being determined to try to do something about them. They needed to help the two older partners bury, if not resolve, their differences as a first step to resolving partnership issues.

Short-term outcome

All partners agreed to meet immediately after the visit. It was an open session to take a rain check on where they were as a group. They discussed whether they should split and rejected that idea. Brian and Calum shook hands and agreed to behave more appropriately and resolve their personal differences outside the practice.

The visit feedback and report had crystallised for Brian and Calum the extent and far-reaching impact of their differences on the practice.

The other partners felt emboldened by the success of this to be more assertive. They pressed for an agreement to a facilitated day out of the practice to take forward the need for a planned and coherent statement of the practice's priorities and values, and a way of deciding on priorities for the way forward. A date for such a day was agreed and the third partner, Fred, was delegated the authority to find a good facilitator. It was felt that given the programme, a highly skilled facilitator was needed to ensure that sensitive and contentious issues were discussed in a non-personal but sensitive way. They further agreed to meet the night before, have a meal and stay overnight. The programme was to include:

- a discussion of values and basic agendas
- a review of current behaviours and practice – what they should start to do and stop doing
- a review of current management arrangements and responsibilities within the partnership, including leadership and chairmanship within the practice
- a plan for the management of the practice in the light of Ella's impending retirement.

The staff were told the gist of the report and the partners' agreed plan of action. They were sceptical about the ability of the partnership to sort itself out, but felt encouraged by the first steps. Following the 'time out', the partners did appear to have undergone some improvements in behaviours and attitudes to each other and the staff. Although there were slips, it was much easier to deal openly with poor or inappropriate spoken or written complaints and grievance, and the practice manager felt emboldened to deal with the miscreants herself.

The staff had a clear list of who was responsible for what and, although they continued to try to manipulate by asking more than one partner for a decision, by and large what the partners wanted was clearer and more understandable. The longer-term planning was still in its infancy, but meetings were chaired and minutes were introduced.

Longer-term outcomes

In the longer term, the partners agreed on a regular day out of the practice, sometimes on their own and sometimes with the practice manager. Once a year they had a practice 'time out' to which everyone came, and the plans for the year were discussed and refined. This was chaired and devised by the practice manager with external facilitators, and was enjoyed by all. The chair of the partnership and the delegated roles within it were reviewed regularly and rotated.

When Ella, the practice manager, finally announced her retirement, the partners' different views on how to replace her threatened to destabilise the practice again. Once more the controlled antagonism between Calum and Brian came to a head. This time they all recognised what was happening and they decided to take the problem out of practice time. At the Saturday afternoon meeting held to discuss the matter, Brian announced that he had decided to take early retirement, so the discussion included the advertising for a new partner.

The practice felt strong and united after this process, and the new practice manager and partner were both excellent. The practice was able to develop its clinical governance role and expand its clinical services to include a nurse practitioner triage. One of the partners became chair of the PCG and subsequently was much involved with the PCT. The regular days out for regaining perspective were seen as essential.

10
Case Study D
Taking time to think

Chapter 2 described the diagnostic consultancy process and Chapters 3–6 discussed in some depth the sort of underlying issues that have been identified over the years and reflected the main ways that have been found to be effective in dealing with specific underlying problems. Tools have been described that can be introduced and a range of questions put, the answers to which can of themselves provoke new ways of thinking and behaving. The aims throughout are always:

- to clarify roles and responsibilities

- to improve people management, including identifying and improving development opportunities for all members of the team

- to increase the awareness and delivery of accountability.

Achievement of all these is predicated on a great commitment to the practice and a will to change. Therefore, over the whole 18 years of our experience there has been one recommendation that has been taken up increasingly and that overrides all the others. That is the need for the practice, the staff team and the partners to take a regular, hard look at themselves and the practice, their philosophy and their management, preferably in a protected time and place, and with external, independent support to manage the process. This is such an important and significant, as well as expensive and disruptive, process that this chapter is devoted to discussing it and incorporates an extended example of one such occasion to illustrate the points made.

One of the commonest cries in practice has been lack of time to stand back, to share aspirations and values with colleagues, to check out assumptions about people's motivations and to share aspirations for the future. Taking time out of the hurly-burly of practice life may be a luxury the practice has always thought they could not afford, but frequently it has proved to be the saving of a partnership and sometimes of the practice as a whole. It has been a way of renewing relationships and of identifying a common path for the future.

The result of inviting an external consultant to review the practice and expose the areas that need attention can be a disturbing and unnerving occasion. Our experience is that it is vital to go to the next stage as quickly as possible. That stage is to digest and consider at leisure and in a relaxed and safe environment what to do about strengthening the areas of weakness and building on the areas of strength revealed. The following background to the case study demonstrates this.

Case Study: Eagle Medical Centre

Background to the 'time out'
The Eagle Medical Centre had invited external consultants to review their practice because they felt they were stagnating and unable to see their way forward. The seven partners (two of them job-sharing) were within a similar age range and had a commonality of view. The staff were well-trained and long-standing with a strong nursing team. The practice manager, Jim, had been at the practice for two years, and was dedicated and energetic. He had, however, been appointed for fundholding and in the light of its demise he was now proposing to retire.

The practice was concerned about how they would replace him. Discussions revealed that the partnership had very divergent views about whether to continue with their experience of strong and effective management or to accept that the new world of PCGs and PCTs meant that practices neither would nor could afford such models. Some partners saw this as an opportunity to stop being so 'leading edge' as a practice with all the change, challenge and disruption that that entailed. Others felt that as the senior partner had not been elected on to the PCG, their interests would be sidelined and a strong practice manager was essential to counter that. The strength of the apparent range of views alarmed them.

The practice had had several previous unproductive 'times out' in the past. Nevertheless, the diagnostic review recommended firmly that the partnership should hold another well-facilitated time out to look at basic values and principles within the partnership. It could establish a baseline from which decisions could be made about the sort of practice they all wanted and the sort of management needed to deliver it. This would provide much-needed time to experience and try out effective ways of testing the views of one's colleagues and one's own assumptions and solutions. It would also provide a safe environment in which to confront any inappropriate behaviour.

After much discussion of the consultants' report, the partners decided that it was imperative that they take the time to think through the internal and external issues affecting the practice. They felt they were at something of a watershed in the practice, and that the investment of a day and a half was a small one in that context.

There are some key issues around the practicalities of such an occasion that can determine its success or failure and therefore need to be resolved before the away day can be arranged. They are as follows:

- the people
- the place
- the aim
- the programme
- facilitation.

The people

The usual core of people present for such an event is the partnership itself, as the partners normally make up the management board and the decision-making team within the practice. If the issues to be discussed are very personal to the partners, they may feel that they do not want anyone from within the practice there to witness such sensitive issues being addressed. Resolving the issue of who should participate can of itself be helpful in freeing up communications within the partnership. Example 45 describes one practice's discussion on the subject.

Example 45

Laundry Lane Surgery had three partners, one of whom, the founder of the practice, owned both the practice premises and a local nursing home at which he spent a great deal of time. His partners were increasingly frustrated at his absence and the consequent high number of locums employed (and paid for) by him, together with his non-appearance at partnership meetings. The other two partners had talked as a duo about excluding him, buying out the premises or offering some other sort of deal, but in very general terms and not coherently. They felt patient care was suffering, certainly the sort of care they wanted to offer from the practice. The practice manager, a friend of the senior partner, provided him with administrative support at the nursing home and so was never party to these discussions.

Eventually, they became so frustrated that they decided to force the issue and use a diagnostic consultant to broker a way forward. The result was a recommendation to take time out with the facilitator to put this, and other thorny problems in the practice, on the table. The partners felt very strongly that the practice manager should not attend the initial away day, because of his role in the nursing home, his rather strong personality and the potentially difficult nature of some of the discussions that were planned for the away day.

Most usually the practice manager is involved in the away day because he or she is intrinsic both to the management of the practice and the way in which most of the decisions made will be implemented. Sometimes the most senior nurse and/or the senior receptionist may be part of a management team and they or others in similar positions may be invited. By and large it is not a good idea to have people coming for only part of the time, as it can create (or reinforce) a feeling of 'them and us'. Where overall practice development is the subject of the time out, it can be helpful to have the whole practice involved, although clearly this is difficult to arrange. Case Study B in Chapter 8 gives an example of what such a whole practice can achieve. The benefits are undoubtedly great if the practice is reasonably small and the group is facilitated in a way that all those present have an equal say and make a contribution.

The Eagle Medical Centre, our case study, had discussions on this issue as well.

Case Study: Eagle Medical Centre

Who to include
There was much discussion over who should attend. Clearly all the part-ners would be there, and there was a general agreement that the practice manager, although he was retiring, would add value. The issue was who else? Some partners felt that the senior nurse and assistant practice manager should be there. The former had been with the practice for ten years and was working at qualifications to be a nurse practitioner. She and the two newest partners envisaged fundamental changes to the nursing role in relation to doctors, and they had even talked about nurse part-ners. However, the partners felt that the presence of the nurse would create unnecessary additional tension.

The assistant practice manager had been running the day-to-day operational side of the practice during the fundholding period and was now hoping to be promoted to the practice manager vacancy. She held the AMGP diploma and was working towards her Diploma in Management Studies. Having talked it through, they all agreed that as her interest in the practice manager's job was public, it would send the wrong message to her if she was invited to join the away day and might inhibit any discussions about the future vacancy.

The last suggestion for additional members was that of the registrar. She had been with the practice for nine months and was very interested in the management side of practice. However, she was finishing her training shortly and the partners decided that although she would undoubtedly get a lot out of the occasion, she would probably add little and possibly would inhibit frank discussion. The registrar was very disappointed in losing out on this opportunity.

The place

There are obvious problems around holding the event in the practice premises – it is almost impossible to ensure no interruptions or people slipping off at breaks to check up on paperwork, make a few phone calls and so on. It is important to have full concentration on the matter in hand and the working environment is not conducive to that because of the possible distractions.

It is also important to be comfortable and have surroundings appropriate to the style of the practice and its way of working. For some practices that may be a boardroom-style conference hotel or centre; for others it may be a comfortable hotel lounge. Whatever the style, it is advisable to provide facilities that show the value the partners place on the occasion and those giving up time to attend. This is particularly true when an overnight or weekend is involved and the practice is therefore encroaching again on personal time. The dinner is, of course, a good way of developing social intercourse, if that is missing, and of starting the event off in a cheerful and convivial way.

The whole arrangement of the event can signal, not just to the partners but also to the staff and the outside world, the level of seriousness with which the practice is taking the issues facing it.

Eagle Medical Centre approached the issue very pragmatically.

> ## Case Study: Eagle Medical Centre
>
> *The place*
> The partners were clear that they wanted a social evening the night before the 'away day', so the event had to be held at a reasonable hotel with a reasonable restaurant to compensate for the time everyone would be spending away from family. Equally, as there would be eight of them they needed a seminar room with separate areas for small groups to work. They chose a local hotel with these facilities and pleasant grounds.

The aim of the time out

The aim of the time out will obviously relate to the findings of the diagnostic consultancy or the perceived needs of the practice. These will vary, but whatever they are they need to be articulated clearly and agreed beforehand. They should be sufficiently clear to share with the rest of the practice, to try to ensure from the start that any feelings of exclusion are limited and the whole practice can share in the outcomes. Example 46 illustrates this.

> ## Example 46
>
> The Bull Street Practice of five partners had felt that they were a very disunited group and put it down to one partner's disruptive behaviour. The problem, as they saw it, was whether to exclude him from the partnership because of this, even though none of them had really confronted him with the problem.
>
> However, the diagnostic visit had revealed deeper variations in views and values across the whole partnership, not just the identified disruptive

partner. The partners appeared to have been unwilling to date to reflect on ways of achieving a common and articulated plan for the future to which all could sign up – doctors, nurses, management and reception staff alike. It appeared that the disruptive partner was being scapegoated and thus excluding him would clearly not be the answer.

The aims of their day out were therefore as follows:

- to share the philosophy and values of the partnership
- to agree the overall way the practice should develop
- to establish priorities for achievement.

Another, different, approach is set out in Example 47.

Example 47

Maud Street Practice, however, had a different approach to their away day because they had a different problem. There were three partners with a close-knit nursing and management team, operating in harmony and very sociably. They presented with unusual and recent high staff turnover and an inability to attract the right calibre and style of person to join the team. The diagnostic visit revealed that the practice was so busy being friendly and sociable that it rarely had the time or inclination to look forward and agree how to achieve plans for the future. In particular, they had not identified opportunities for members of the team to take on new responsibilities within the practice, within the PCG and in the wider professional world, whatever that might be.

The aims for the day out therefore were as follows:

- to identify future needs, opportunities and potential development for the practice
- to enable individuals to identify personal, educational and developmental needs in that context.

Our case study practice, Eagle Medical Centre, illustrates that it is a good idea to start the formal sessions of the time out by putting on the table the participants' expectations of the day and the individual priorities for achievement for the day.

Case Study: Eagle Medical Centre

The aim of the day

Initially, it was thought to be a simple matter to define the aim of the day. However, it became clear in discussion that although all partners wanted 'to find a way forward' there were differing views as to how this would be achieved. David saw the day as a structured and formal way of agreeing a business plan for the next year. Martin saw it as a way of talking through the current workload issues. The others, Fiona, Catherine, Len, John and Phillip, saw it as a way of getting out issues that they had bottled up for years. It was agreed that the facilitators would circulate a short question-naire to all those attending, one purpose of which would be to define the expectations of the day, and from which they would prepare a draft for everyone to approve.

The facilitators also suggested that the questionnaire, which would be confidential between the individual and the facilitator, should ask one or two other questions about personal motivation and priorities that would help them plan the day.

Confidential

Outline of confidential questionnaire for Eagle Medical Centre Partners

Please complete the following and return to the facilitator:

1 My expectations of the day:
   - for myself
   - for the partnership
   - for the practice

2 Three significant reasons why I work

3 What I value most about general practice and what gives me most job satisfaction

4 My top three priorities for the practice in next three years

From the answers to Question 1 the facilitators summarised the aims of the day as being:

- to gain greater knowledge and understanding of partners' aims and ambitions
- to improve decision making in the practice.

It was agreed that if these aims were achieved, the immediate issues, such as how to replace the practice manager, and others concerning the amount of time spent out of the practice by partners, and the training practice status could be tackled sensibly and coherently. Unless the underlying causes of conflict were addressed in a focused way, there would be no long-term ways imbedded for dealing with difficult and/or contentious issues that might arise in the future.

The programme

The programme for the day needs to be ambitious but realistic, moving carefully but firmly from the general and safe, where agreement is likely, to the more specific and less safe, where agreement will be more difficult to achieve. It is sometimes useful for partners to write down individually their ideas for the day and for the programme to be compiled from an amalgam of those ideas.

A useful starting point is to agree ground rules of behaviour for the day, a suggested list of which is given in Box 10.1.

Box 10.1: Ground rules

1 What happens today will be confidential to the group except for the issues/decisions the group agrees to reveal to others.
2 The task or objectives will be clear and agreed before the discussions begin.
3 Discussion will be pertinent to the task.
4 Everyone will listen to each other.
5 Everyone will be prepared to give examples to support statements and opinions.
6 Criticism will be frank, constructive and non-personal, and be about what people do, not what they are.

7 The group will be as open as possible and differences of opinion will be respected.

8 Differences will be expressed, not suppressed, and false consensus will be avoided; if there is disagreement, the group will seek to resolve the differences, not ignore them.

9 The key decision of the day regarding the contract will be made by consensus, not majority rule. Other decisions will also be made by consensus rather than majority rule, wherever possible.

10 When action is agreed, roles will be assigned and accepted.

11 The group will monitor its own progress and stop frequently to examine how well it is doing or what may be interfering with its operation.

12 The facilitator's roles will be clear and agreed.

It is often helpful to design a programme that gives opportunities throughout the day to break into twos and threes. This enables people to work closely together on an issue and to support each other in presenting and selling their conclusions to the whole group.

The aim should always be to have agreed a plan of action by the end of the time, and to finish on a high note, hence the careful planning of the programme. The case study shows how this can work in one instance.

Case Study: Eagle Medical Centre

The programme for the day

09.00	Introduction	Plenary
09.15	Ground rules for the day agreed	Plenary
	Facilitators' role to be explained and agreed	Plenary
09.30	Expectations of the day discussed and agreed	Plenary
09.45	Common and dissimilar motivations	Small groups
	(based on pre-away day questionnaire)	
	Common themes	Plenary
	(chaired by a partner)	

10.45	Coffee	
11.00	Values	Small groups
	(based on pre-away day questionnaire)	
	Common themes	Plenary
	(chaired by another partner)	
12.00	Where do I want the practice to be in three years' time?	Small groups
	(based on pre-away day questionnaire)	
	Common themes and agreed aims	
Plenary		
	(chaired by another partner)	
13.00	Lunch	
14.00	Helps and obstacles to achieving the agreed aims	Small groups
	Common themes	Plenary
	(chaired by another partner)	
14.45	What to stop, start and continue doing	
	(chaired by another partner)	
15.30	Tea	
15.45	Action plan	Plenary
	(chaired by another partner)	

Facilitation

Running such a time out can be a complex and testing task. A good facilitator with all the skills required of such a role, someone not involved in the issues under discussion and with no particular axe to grind could make the difference between a successful day and a disaster. Without a facilitator someone within the partnership will need to chair the day. They will be inhibited from participating fully, not least because of the chair's responsibilities to keep the debate flowing, protecting those under attack and making sure the timetable is moved through at a reasonable pace. This is very difficult for a practice manager to do, not least because the nature of the employer/employee relationship must inhibit the firmness with which facilitation sometimes needs to be exercised. The practice manager

Box 10.2: Facilitator's role

- To help the group perceive, understand and act on the day in order to achieve the aims of the afternoon.
- To provide knowledge and expertise when necessary.
- To help the group clarify issues, by encouraging the group to analyse and conclude from their experiences.
- To help the members of the group consider the consequences of their behaviour.
- To reflect back observations and impressions to the group.
- To be non-directive.
- To test consensus.
- To remind the group of the ground rules when necessary.
- To help the group handle conflict if it arises.
- To keep the group to time.

would be in an invidious position if the facilitation demands firmness in handling confrontation or blockage between partners, or partners and staff.

A trusted facilitator can make all the difference to time out, particularly if they have some knowledge of the practice, ideally from a diagnostic visit. In that way they will be aware of the hidden agendas and the personality traits of the people involved and can exercise their neutral role more confidently. Box 10.2 gives a list of the tasks for an external facilitator, which need to be agreed by the group before the day starts.

With all these factors well sorted out and agreed beforehand, the protected time out of the practice is one of the healthiest and most productive uses of time a practice can invest. Eagle Medical Centre demonstrates this.

Case Study: Eagle Medical Centre

The away day
The pre-away day dinner. The dinner the night before the away day was a great success. The seven partners, the practice manager and the

two facilitators had a relaxed and convivial time, discussing their interests and families, the world situation and the state of the health services, without specifically discussing anything related directly to the practice.

Introductory session. The next morning started rather stiffly, but the introduction helped to establish where everybody had come from. The facilitators reminded the group of the main conclusions of the diagnostic consultancy report:

- to check common values and priorities within the partnership
- to plan for the future
- to improve decision making and chairing
- to confront inappropriate behaviour.

They explained that the programme of the day was not just about working through the issues, but also for the partners to practise effective decision-making and chairing skills. This would also give opportunities to criticise and confront assertively but positively, and for the group to reflect on its own teamworking. Each plenary session was therefore to be chaired by a different partner, and time was set aside at the end of each session to reflect back on the quality of the chairing, the decision making as a group process and the supportiveness of the team.

At the end of each session the person chairing would be first asked to reflect on:

- how they felt
- where they thought they did well in chairing the discussion and less well
- what they thought the decision was
- if the outcome was unanimous.

The group was then asked to reflect on whether:

- the chair had enabled the discussion to progress
- the chair had ensured everyone could be heard
- the chair had ensured everyone voiced their views
- the chair checked understanding and consensus at each stage in the discussion
- the chair had summarised and got agreement at the end.

First session. The first session on motivation was reasonably light-hearted and the two groups came together well. The object of the plenary session was to come to an agreement as a group as to the similarities and dissimilarities between partners. Martin, who was chairing, set out the purpose of the session and got each group to report back their views. He then tended to let the discussion drift because he had an interest in a particular line. He used 'I' a great deal, rather than encouraging others to give an opinion. He spoke more than anyone else did. He showed no insight into this, but thought he enabled people to speak and express views. He thought he had not summed up well, but had identified the questions that the session had not resolved and got these on a separate flip chart for resolution later.

The group was very encouraging and supportive, and made no criticisms of his style or the way the discussion had gone. They felt they had revealed things about each other that they had not known and that these would help in understanding problems that occurred over decisions.

The facilitators were supportive but pointed out some of the less effective elements in his chairing style, concentrating on quoting actual things that had happened in the discussion and the actual recorded number percentage of time that Martin spoke out of the total discussion time, namely 45%. The partners agreed that it had been difficult to get a word in and that the chair had been intent on going along one particular route. The facilitators then asked why none of the partners had pointed this out. They agreed that it was because they did not want to upset the partner concerned and were anxious for others not to criticise them when their turn came. This was where inability to address real issues of difference and conflict came from – fear and 'there but for the grace of God' attitude, which was ultimately unhelpful both to the partnership and the practice.

Second session. The group now knew more about what got them where they were and why. The second session about values was much more hard-hitting, with the small groups getting down to identifying those things that each held most dear in their work. The small groups had to identify three common values they shared and the three most significant differences.

The facilitators asked Peter to chair the plenary session. Again, the object was to come to some agreement as a group as to the similarities and dissimilarities of the partnership value system.

Peter had very clear views on his values and was at one end of the spectrum that emerged from the presentation of the two groups. He was unable to stand back from the discussion but kept interjecting as others presented their views. Although he stated the purpose of the session and made clear what he expected as the outcome, he did not get the group to agree except on the superficialities. The facilitators had to step in and probe the group. They revealed really fundamental differences between those who saw the practice as remaining at the leading edge of practice at all costs and those who were happy to be an average general practice, giving good care and keeping a reasonable balance between home and work.

The review of the process afterwards was much sharper. Peter realised from the facilitators' interventions how he had failed to draw out the real differences between the partners. The rest of the group spoke their minds about his style and their resentment of the way he conducted the meeting. The facilitators therefore went on to ask the group why they had not said how they felt to the chair during the meeting. He might have found it helpful and they could have negotiated a different style. They all agreed.

Third session. The third session on priorities for the practice was well-chaired by Fiona. She checked understanding and kept the group to the task. She made helpful suggestions to prioritise the wide range of priorities brought by the small groups into the plenary. She suggested that they sort them into the priorities under the different areas of the practice's life:

- clinical/patient services
- education
- research
- management
- finance
- patient services
- external relations
- quality assurance/clinical governance.

As a result the group ended up with clear priorities within each head and a list of other action points to be discussed later.

The feedback on chairing was very positive, much to the obvious surprise of the chair and the group itself, as she had never been seen as a natural leader of the group. They had all related chairing skills to leadership. The fact that one could be detached from the other was a revelation. This session overran into lunch and the group decided to cut the length of lunch and still start at 14.00 for the afternoon session.

Fourth session. The session on the obstacles to achieving the aims went well in small groups. They were asked to look at the broad priorities agreed and identify what had to happen to achieve them, including things that had to stop, things that must start and things that should continue. In order to try to ensure that all the areas were covered, the two small groups divided the priorities between them.

The feedback session was chaired by the least confident of the partners, Phillip, and very soon the two most vociferous and dynamic, Martin and John, took the process over. The first small group, which contained both these partners, went through their priorities carefully. They had flip charts for each.

Eagle Medical Centre Priority 1

Improved decision making in the partnership – Action plan
STOP

- making assumptions about the meaning of silence
- being intransigent
- confusing leadership with chairing skills

START

- listening
- stroking each other positively
- having a proactive approach to meetings – read minutes, prepare agendas with background papers
- review decision making – should it be by veto, unanimous only or consensus
- review chairmanship of meetings

CONTINUE

- listening
- pushing and encouraging from senior partner

They were very pleased with themselves and were not very interested in listening to the work from the other small group, and Phillip was not able to bring them to order. There was a lot of muttering and grumbling in the ranks until one of the facilitators asked the first group how they were planning to do the things they had suggested. This provoked a silence and then everyone started to talk at once as to ways in which some of the behavioural changes could be made.

The facilitators decided to stop the discussion and talk about the decision-making and chairing process. Phillip was very depressed because he felt he had lost it from the word go and could not get control of the key players. The others agreed that that was the case and that the process was therefore shambolic. The facilitators asked whether the rest of the group felt they had any responsibility for the process or was it all down to the chair? The vociferous partner said that that was what a chair was there to do – to control the group. Catherine said that perhaps the group had some responsibilities to control itself. Fiona – as light dawned – said that she should have helped Phillip by joining with him in trying to show Martin and John what they were doing to the process. There was silence. And then Phillip said that he had felt let down by the group and alone, and would have welcomed some support. The others all agreed that they had behaved badly in their various ways, both actively and passively, and all apologised for their shortcomings. The second group was then able to go through its charts and add in the 'how' column.

Action plan. By now the closing time was fast approaching and it was not possible to complete all the priorities. All agreed, however, that they had got the idea of the method and would go away and finish it, perhaps with the rest of the management group, even with the rest of the practice. The facilitators pointed out that even though time was short, it was essential to agree an action plan for the next stage, however limited that might be. They therefore identified the next key actions, which were:

- to feed back to the rest of the team the key outcomes of the day
- to set an agenda for a practice team away day, which could be based on the priorities list they had drawn up
- to have a partnership meeting to talk through the away day, especially the issues around personal behaviours and the chair of the partnership

- to expect a report of the day from the facilitators which would form the basis for both the away day with the managers and the next steps.

Review of the day. The last few minutes of the away day were taken up with concentration on a review of the day. They discussed whether their expectations had been reached and agreed that their expectations had been unrealistic but that the day had identified ways for meeting their expectations in the future. The positives were that they had largely kept to time, which was a major thing for the practice, they had focused on the task in hand, they had stayed out of the practice and they had kept going. They had also got better and more constructive at challenging each other and occasionally the facilitators!

They were taking away a much greater understanding of each other's motivations and agendas in life as well as the practice. They also all felt more confident at confronting each other and of chairing effectively. All had gained some insights into their own strengths and weaknesses, and all committed themselves to being open with each other about them. They also had a strong feel for the real priorities, the sticking points and the options facing them. They were all clear that they wished to go forward together and to find ways of working together in spite of their differences of ways of operating and priorities. They felt they were stronger together than apart – the real meaning of teams.

Longer-term outcomes. The partnership had a series of partnership meetings – on Saturday afternoons and evenings – to work thorough the rest of the priorities. They then shared those priorities with the practice team and had a full meeting of the practice to take on board any suggestions. Several amendments were made as a result. Jim agreed to stay on for another year while the partnership and practice sorted out their priorities. The partners had another day out (unfacilitated) specifically to draw up a job description for the practice manager's replacement, and found that they were able to agree almost without debate on the level of delegation they were looking for. The new practice manager, Julie, was appointed after an extensive recruitment and selection process that included the use of an external assessor.

At the end of the year they were clear as a partnership and a practice as to their priorities, and they had a new practice manager who had a clear job description and a good understanding of the practice values and philosophy. They were also much more aware of the need for good chairing of meetings, good and effective leadership on the various elements of practice life, and the means of dealing with divergences within the partnership. They agreed on regular, facilitated away days every year to ensure this progress was maintained.

Part 4
The future

11
Where now?

Many general practice organisations appear to be under siege in the modern NHS, barely coping with demands being made upon them and unable to stand back and take a strategic view of the needs of GPs (Marshall, 1999). However, this book has also shown how many practices have come to grips with difficult, immediate issues as well as begun to develop strategies and plans for improving underlying situations.

Accommodating the future changes and developments that will undoubtedly come will be more successful if the lessons of the past and the present are used both as a springboard and as a means of gaining confidence in approaching the challenges that undoubtedly lie ahead.

We have seen that the main problems besetting practice, underlying all the presenting issues of time, workload, inadequate personnel, insufficient resources and so on, fall within the four headings of:

- common values and philosophies
- management awareness
- working across boundaries
- accountability.

These key messages tie in with the two most important developments facing general practice today. The first is the structural and organisational one, namely, PCGs (and their Scottish and Welsh equivalents) and their successor bodies. The second is increased accountability and patient-focused care, through the twin developments of state-driven clinical govern- ance and professionally-driven revalidation of the licence to practice, both based on forms of regular appraisal.

PCGs, LHBs and LHCs enhance the message that good management is at the heart of good clinical care. Indeed, the two crucial requirements for the success of these bodies and their successful translation to PCT status in England have been identified in a study of the progress of the PCGs, LHBs and LHCs by the Health Services Management Centre in Birm- ingham as 'effective clinical leadership ... and the quality of general management support available'. In turn, public trust and accountability rely on good systems to demonstrate appropriate efforts to produce best outcomes in a judgement-based science such as medicine. Our experience demonstrates what the keys to developing such expertise and culture really are and how they can unlock the real potential of general practice and its role in developing primary care.

The organisational demands of the future

All the management and organisational skills that this book has addressed will be in demand in the new organisational and commissioning role demanded by the new structures. Identify- ing common goals and visions, acquiring and maintaining high- level management skills, working across more boundaries than in a single practice and dealing with a range of accountabilities will be the name of the game at whatever level of involvement a practice places itself.

The PCG/LHC/LHG structure will require board members to demonstrate a corporate approach rather than appear to repre- sent individual professions or geographical groups. Indeed, it is vital that PCGs corporately and their individual stakeholders feel that they have been actively consulted and are committed to taking forward plans and actions which will implement HImP priorities. PCGs should be uniquely placed to ensure that evidence of local healthcare needs and the views of clinicians and their patients are reflected in local HImPs. Individual GPs and nurses too will need to feed into this and provide the essential and comprehensive data, staff, skills, service and facilities currently held within practice, but as we have seen (Chapters 4 and 6) not always available from it.

> No one agency or staff is likely to be able to achieve all that is being asked of PCGs on their own. Successful PCGs will be those that can harness the range of skills necessary to learn and work together for an effective partnership which will improve patient care.

The message here is training, training, training.

The NHS Plan flags changes to the status of GPs as the use of PMS pilots (formally PCAPS) is expanded, for example, in allowing the appointment of salaried doctors, that is GPs working outside the standard terms and conditions of service. Throughout there will be greater focus on the needs of patients, and doctors will need to understand more clearly the distribution of the power ratios within the PCT (Chapter 3). The next step, that of PCT status, will bring added freedoms and opportunities to develop but at the expense of greater risks and uncertainties (Callaghan *et al.*, 2000).

Partnerships

The whole concept of working across boundaries will expand as localised collaboration becomes a necessary part of the complex set of relationships in health and social care. 'Collaborative advantage will be achieved when something unusually creative is produced ... that no organisation could have produced on its own and when each organisation, through collaboration, is able to achieve its own objectives better than it could alone' (Huxham, 1993). GPs are now in the majority on PCG boards and as such will be expected to bring together a range of organisations and professions, each with their own interests and constituencies, to develop an effective partnership in commissioning and providing primary healthcare. Their experience within the practice will be a springboard for this sort of development (Chapter 5), as long as the time and money are available for the acquisition of the vital skills.

Planning

The new HImPs are generating enthusiasm at a local level. They are three-year local plans intended to bring together main statutory and voluntary bodies in each health authority area, including housing, transport, education and employment, to plan and deliver means to improve the health of the local population. However, extending ownership and maintaining commitment are necessary if they are to deliver reduced inequalities and better health, and working in partnership is a core element of HImP development. As we have demonstrated, clarity of vision and roles is vital in such situations. It is of concern that when many practices are still coming to grips with strategic planning, PCGs tend to be dominated by GPs. Tangible improvements must be delivered or the expanded partnership working will rapidly descend into meaningless bureaucracy and the whole concept of working together will be harmed.

Accountability

Accountability underpins the collaborative culture necessary for clinical governance to work. As we have seen (Chapter 6), clinical governance represents a collaborative contract between government, NICE, and local managers and professionals. It will also reflect the user needs, although the transparency sought by patients does not always coincide with state expediency and parliamentary convenience. Clinical governance will need to establish the primacy of the individual professional's collaborative obligation to their organisation, their patients and the public before their loyalty to professional colleagues (Dewar, 2000).

In the terms of the Audit Commission report (1999), clinical governance embraces for primary care:

- agreeing clear standards and responsibilities
- multidisciplinary clinical audit and follow-up
- improving quality of clinical data
- supporting evidence-based practice and implementation of quality guidelines
- dissemination of good practice
- dealing with poor practice
- ensuring that adverse events are investigated and lessons applied
- programmes to reduce risk.

Marshall (1999) identified seven barriers that health authorities face as they manage quality improvement in general practice in the context of NHS reforms. They are very similar to those identified in this book.

- The absence of an explicit strategic plan.
- Competing priorities for the attention of the directors.
- The sensitivity of health professionals.

- A lack of information due to poor-quality clinical data.

- A lack of authority to implement change.

- Unclear roles and responsibilities of managers in the organisation.

- The isolation of managers from other organisations facing similar challenges.

The risk of using performance management to drive progress is that the very people who are meant to be delivering it lose ownership of health improvement. There is a balance to be struck between orders issued from the centre that need to be followed rigidly and those that allow local flexibility. The much-needed increased investment in the NHS, beginning to compensate for long years of starvation of new funds, is presented as an incentive to plan and produce effective change, but carries with it very powerful threats of reparation if the priority improvements are not demonstrated.

Those factors make the increased professional accountability required by professionally driven revalidation all the more important (RCGP, 2000b). Removing the public and professional perception that registration as a doctor is a ticket for life is an important step in this direction. It gives the profession enhanced confidence in its skills and professionalism, gives the public confidence in the skills and relevance of a doctor's qualifications, and parallels the state's increased used of its contractual tools to demand and monitor standards and service.

Professional occupations possess:

- a systematic body of highly developed technical knowledge that is widely valued

- strong standards of autonomy that emphasise self-regulation and altruism that submerge self-interest and emphasise service

- a need for extensive authority over clients
- a distinct occupational culture and collegial etiquette
- recognition of this professional status by political, social and economic leadership (Rosenthal, 1999).

Having to demonstrate the above (particularly the first) to peers and lay people in a regular way strengthens the relationship between public and profession. That relationship is very strong – the majority of the British public (81% in relation to GPs) agrees that the medical profession in general keeps up to date with the knowledge required to practice their profession (Corrado and Marett, 1999). But to maintain and enhance that position will require the further acquisition and use of those skills and insights, which we have identified in this book as underlying the problems of past practice. As we have noted, it needs development, offered in a participative and authoritative setting, so that doctors can transfer their clinical skills to management and organisational issues. This assertion is based on our experience of training and developing in small groups with GPs and practice managers (Huntingdon and Irvine, 1992), general practice trainers (Haman and Irvine, 1998a) and GPs in small groups (Haman and Irvine, 1998b). Indeed, they are increasingly able to see that often there is little clear water between them.

And where now?

In this country, we appear in many ways to distrust our doctors more and are increasingly cynical about the potential of the medical system. In Porter's words, 'There is an unresolved dis-equilibrium between the remarkable capacity of the increasingly powerful, science-based biomedical tradition, and the wider and unfulfilled health requirements of economically impoverished, colonially vanquished and politically mismanaged societies.' This makes it tough for those who are the inheritors of the one and the physicians of the other. However, it is clear that only the public, the government, the NHS and the health professions *together* can achieve the order of quality that should become the norm for a new millennium (Irvine, 1999).

The good news is that patients prefer smaller practices if they can form mutually supportive confederations that offer traditional patient care together with advantages in terms of services and divisions of responsibilities of larger practices (Dixon, 2000). A mixed economy of salaried and independent contractors holding a generalist role will be increasingly in demand as secondary care specialisation continues unabated. This seems a good outcome for the individual GP and for patients.

Corporate governance and enhanced professional performance review in primary care will create a new culture of change, improve average standards and reduce lower standards of care. There will be a new balance between hard clinical evidence and holistic forces, cultural trends and tradition. These will help to restore the level of trust from patients previously enjoyed by the medical profession.

In this book we have drawn on the experiences of a large number of practices. The teams working within and around those practices have built on their strengths, faced up to their difficulties and deficiencies, and tried out a range of solutions to show that general practice in the primary and intermediate care setting can rise to these new demands.

Using the lessons from those experiences and examples will help all those concerned with delivering high-quality primary and community care to meet effectively the ever-increasing expectations of patients and the demands for greater accountability and demonstration of value for money from the government. It will help balance the potential of developing technologies with the traditional values of care, and manage the continuing uncertainty about the structure and institutions within which that care is delivered. These are significant challenges for all involved.

References

Arora S, Davies A and Thompson S (2000) Challenges for a new millennium. *J Interprof Care.* **14**.

Audit Commission (1999) *The PCG Agenda: early progress of PCGs in England.* The Stationery Office, London.

Bloor K, Maynard A and Street A (1999) *The Cornerstone of Labour's New NHS: reforming primary care.* Centre for Health Education, York.

Bosanquet N and Leese B (1989) *Family Doctors and Economic Incentives.* Dartmouth Publishing Co, Aldershot.

Callaghan G *et al.* (2000) Prospects for collaboration in primary care: relationships between social services and the new PCGs. *J Interprof Care.* **14**.

Carlisle S, Elwyn G and Smail S (2000) Personal and practice development plans in primary care in Wales. *J Interprof Care.* **14**.

Chief Medical Officer of England (1998) *Review of Continuing Professional Development in General Practice.* The Stationery Office, London.

Corrado M and Marett S (1999) *Attitudes Towards Doctors and Their Code of Conduct.* Research study conducted for SCHARR/University of Sheffield and UCL on behalf of the GMC. GMC, London.

Department of Health (1989) *Working for Patients.* HMSO, London.

Department of Health (1990) *The New Contract.* HMSO, London.

Department of Health (1996a) *Choices and Opportunities.* The Stationery Office, London.

Department of Health (1996b) *A Service With Ambition*. The Stationery Office, London.

Department of Health (1997) *The New NHS: modern, dependable*. The Stationery Office, London.

Department of Health (2000) *The NHS Plan*. The Stationery Office, London.

Dewar S (2000) Collaborating for quality: the need for a strong backbone of accountability. *J Interprof Care*. **14**.

Dixon M (2000) Co-operative working relationships. *J Interprof Care*. **14**.

Elwyn G and Smail S (1998) *Personal and Practice Development Plans in Primary Care*. University of Wales College of Medicine, School of Postgraduate Medical and Dental Education, Cardiff.

General Medical Council (1995) *Duties of a Doctor: good medical practice*. GMC, London.

Haman H and Irvine S (1998a) Appraisal for general practice development: an evaluation of a programme of appraisal courses held in the Northern Region 1995/6. *Edu Gen Prac*. **9**: 44–50.

Haman H and Irvine S (1998b) Management support for audit. *Audit Trends*. **6**: 27–9.

Haman H and Irvine S (1997) *Making Sense of Personnel Management* (2e). Radcliffe Medical Press, Oxford.

Haman H and Irvine S (2001) *Good Practice, Good People: a practical guide to managing personnel in the new primary care organisations*. Radcliffe Medical Press, Oxford.

Heifetz D (1997) The work of leadership. *HBR*. **Jan/Feb**.

Hertzberg F (1966) *Work and the Nature of Man*. World Publishing, New York.

Huntingdon J and Irvine S (1992) *Management Appreciation: the book*. RCGP, London.

Huxham T (1993) Pursuing collaborative advantage. *J Oper Res Soc*. **44**(6): 599–611.

Irvine D (1999) *The Performance of Doctors: quality, accountability and the public interest*. The Harben Lecture (unpublished).

Irvine D and Irvine S (1996) *The Practice of Quality*. Radcliffe Medical Press, Oxford (out of print).

Jelley D (1999) *Peer Appraisal*. Unpublished doctorate assignment, University of Newcastle.

Jelley D (2000) *Management Systems and Personnel*. Unpublished doctorate assignment, University of Newcastle.

Kotter JP (1990) *What Leaders Really Do*. Harvard Business School Press, Boston.

Marks L and Hunter DJ (1998) *The Development of PCGs: policy into practice*. The NHS Federation, London.

Marshall M (1999) Improving quality in general practice: qualitative assessment of barriers faced by health authorities. *BMJ*. **319**: 164–7.

Mintzberg H (1980) *The Nature of Managerial Work*. Prentice-Hall, New York.

Northumberland Health Authority (1999) Personal communication.

Øvretveit J (1992) *Health Service Quality*. Blackwell Scientific Publications, Oxford.

RCGP (1999) *Good Medical Practice for General Practice: report of the GMP Working Party*. RCGP, London.

RCGP (2000a) *Evolving Accountability in General Practice*. Consultation document. RCGP, London.

RCGP (2000b) *Revalidation for General Practitioners: criteria, standards and evidence*. Consultation document. RCGP, London.

Robbins H and Finley M (1997) *Why Teams Don't Work*. Orion Business Books, London.

Roland M and Baker R (1999) *Clinical Governance: a practical guide for primary care teams*. University of Manchester, Manchester.

Rosenthal MM (1999) How doctors think about medical mishaps. In: MM Rosenthal, L Mulcahy and S Lloyd-Bostock (eds) *Medical Mishaps: pieces of the puzzle*. Open University Press, Buckingham.

Salter B (1999) *Who Rules? The new politics of medical regulation*. University of East Anglia (Unpublished).

Teal T (1996) The human side of management. *HBR*. **Nov/Dec**.
Zaleznik A (1977) Managers and leaders: are they different?
  HBR. **May/June**.

Further reading

Adair J (1988) *Effective Leadership*. Pan, London.
Department of Health (1999) *Clinical Governance: quality and the
  NHS*. The Stationery Office, London.
Department of Health (1999) *Continuous Professional Devel-
  opment: quality in the new NHS*. The Stationery Office,
  London.
General Medical Council (2000) *Revalidation for Doctors*. GMC,
  London.
Health Service Management Centre (2000) *A Study of the
  Progress of PCGs, LHBs, and LHCCs*. HSMC, Birmingham.
Klein R and Dixon J (2000) Cash bonanza for NHS. *BMJ*. **320**:
  883–4.
RCGP (1998) *Quality Practice Award*. RCGP, London.
Syder B and Tofts A (1999) *The Phoenix Agenda: a development
  framework for primary care group leaders*. NHS Executive/NHS
  Confederation, London.
Whiteman J (2000) Inter-professional education: the challenge
  to GP education in the light of the new NHS. *J Interprof
  Care*. **14**.
van Zwanenburg T and Harrison J (eds) (2000) *Clinical Govern-
  ance in Primary Care*. Radcliffe Medical Press, Oxford.

Appendix A
What is diagnostic consultancy?

There are five main elements.

1 A pre-visit discussion with a consultant gauges the range of issues on which the practice seeks help and therefore the range of interviews that will be needed. Usually, the consultant will have a long telephone discussion with the commissioner about the reasons for the visit to get an idea of the practice, its size and complexity, and the people involved. A rough estimate of time and process will be given and a letter sent confirming the proposed arrangements.

The plan is usually to timetable in as many members of the whole team as possible for interview. From this early discussion the consultant can judge the likely length of the visit (typically two days actually interviewing and two days' preparation and report writing) plus any material required beforehand. This material usually includes the practice leaflet, a recent annual report, the business plan, a staff organisation chart and a list of personnel. These are sent to the consultant and a draft timetable of interviews is produced at this point.

2 The visit is then arranged, if possible over two consecutive days and ending on the second day with a meeting with all partners to give early feedback. This is the key part of the process as it is through the actual visit that the consultants have the opportunity to develop relationships with all concerned, gain trust and confidence, and establish what is really going on in the practice.

It is usually helpful to start with a tour of the premises and an introductory talk with the commissioning partner or practice manager. This first interview is important as it sets the tone of the visit and gives the widest sweep of the practice. Therefore, it is vital that the first interviewee is someone who is likely to get something out of the visit and is not silent or resistant. As a rule of thumb, all partners are interviewed wherever possible for at least an hour and the practice manager, where appointed, similarly. Other staff interviews range in time between 15 and 30 minutes depending on length of service and pertinence to the presenting problem.

Confidentiality is stressed at all times. Nothing will be attributed without consent. This is very important because in a short time it is vital that people feel able to say what they feel and want in a safe environment.

Interviews, particularly the longer ones, are in-depth and concentrate as much on discussing the views and ideas of the partners or senior staff as collecting information.

3 The interviews have a major developmental purpose, as the consultant attempts to help the interviewee to look at the positive aspects of the practice, as well as at its problems, from different viewpoints. It can be an opportunity to test an interviewee's standpoint. Often the interviewee may recite the accepted view of a situation but under gentle probing may come to see that they are starting from the wrong standpoint or misunderstanding the situation. Often the interviews are an opportunity to establish an awareness of the management capacity of the interviewee and their training needs.

But the interviews are also fact-finding and it is important to test statements by one interviewee with another, to check the nature of the view. Is it a significant view based on fact or an individual moan, a bitter reaction to a bad event, a personal vendetta or a personal flag-waving exercise?

Issues discussed may include:

- the nature and location of the leadership function within the practice, how decisions are made
- the motivational needs of partners and staff (and everyone's awareness of them)
- the ability of the practice (particularly the partnership) to confront difficult issues (such as an aggressive partner, an inadequate practice manager, a bullying receptionist, a rigid practice nurse)
- how much is delegated effectively to whom and why.

The aim is to ensure that the feedback session at the end of the visit holds no surprises for the partners individually or together. So it is important to gain consent from the interviewee at the end of the interview as to what can be fed back in an attributable way and what has to remain anonymous. If the latter, it sometimes means it is lost for good if only that interviewee can have made that particular point. Sometimes, however, if for instance a group of nurses have a common view, it is possible to put it forward, as no one individual is recognisable.

After the interviews the consultants consider all that has been said and align it to their experience of practices and background information obtained to come to a diagnosis of the underlying problems.

4 The verbal feedback is given at the end of the visit, desirably to all partners. It reflects back the consultants' immediate impressions and gives key analyses. In this session it is important to be concise and clear, and to concentrate on a few key messages. It is important to reflect back as quickly as possible on the issues that have arisen in the interviews. At this stage in the consultancy, people are still reflecting on the new ways of looking at old issues that the interviews may have provided. The verbal feedback helps to build on the confidence to challenge shibboleths that have gone unchallenged and can help develop self-confidence and assertiveness among some that have been squashed up until now by stronger and more aggressive partners.

It is also the opportunity to let partners be open with each other – often for the first time – and to articulate things previously left unspoken but revealed in the one-to-one interviews. The wider experience of other practices visited and the wider national scene is often an important ingredient both in gaining credibility and in widening the horizons of those who inevitably have been somewhat blinkered in their concerns for the apparently insurmountable problems which they are trying to overcome.

Usually the feedback begins with giving thanks to the usually considerable effort that has gone into making the visit comfortable and effective. The consultant then reflects on the strengths of the practice to ensure that the analysis of where things can be improved is cushioned on a bed of comfort. It is frequent for partners in particular to be very hard on themselves and their colleagues and it is important to ensure that the balance is right. The consultants then usually set the context of the areas where the practice might want to concentrate its efforts at improvement. Recommendations as to the options for the way forward are offered.

Usually practices have so much to absorb at that stage that the discussion of the verbal feedback is limited. The consultants often leave so that the partners can discuss the key highlights among themselves. Alternatively, the partners are sometimes eager to understand more fully what is going on and/or want to fix the next steps immediately.

5 A full written report follows within two weeks, which reinforces the messages of the feedback session. It is written in a way that can be read by all the key players and a précis might be included that is less sensitive and can be shown to others in the team.

Appendix B
Practice strengths

The following are some examples of factors that can indicate strengths.

Partners

- The partnership has been together a long time.

- The partnership is a young, dynamic group.

- The partners may have strong social bonds and close family connections.

- The partnership group meets frequently.

- There are strong professional bonds and a common approach.

- The partners appear to trust each other clinically and share values in relation to the focus of the practice – doctor or patient.

- There is a shared attitude to new developments such as fundholding, and nowadays PCGs.

- The practice team shares a common interest in validation internally and externally through, for instance, being a training practice or seeking to obtain the accreditation of IIP or FbA.

- Members of the team who are interested in contributing to wider professional matters through involvement in, for instance, their professional asssociation or PCG development are supported.

- The practice supports those members of the team who are interested in developing new areas of interest or gaining additional qualifications and expertise.

- A value has been agreed on the contribution external activities have for the practice.

- There is a common pool for income, at least between partners.

- There is authentic agreement by the partnership as to the distribution of fees from external activities.

Policies

- The practice has regular meetings, which are open and clear in their analysis of issues. They are chaired effectively and have explicit agendas, agreed and complete minutes, and make tangible and measurable decisions.

- The practice decision-making process reflects regular audits, which ensure the decisions are made on sustainable data.

- There is a systematic approach ensuring the practice both knows what it is doing and can identify areas needing improvement.

- There are clear policies about patient access and the use of consultations, by doctor or nurse.

- The nursing team is extensively used and managed.

- IT is effectively integrated within the team.

The practice manager

- The practice manager is loyal and long-serving, knowing the patients well, and is known and trusted by them.

- The practice manager has been promoted from the reception team and is trusted and respected by them.

- The practice manager has come from outside the practice and has become established through his/her knowledge and skills with the staff and patients.

- They are hardworking and have saved – or made – the practice money in terms of time and potential litigation.

- They have contributed to the ideas and development of the practice.

- They have a positive attitude to problems, always turning a 'can't do' into 'a can do' situation.

- They are interested in developing their skills and the skills of others through wider external experiences such as with AMGP [now The Institute of Healthcare Management (IHM)] and/or the development of commissioning and HImPs.

Management expertise

- The partners have delegated areas of practice activity to named partners and the practice manager or equivalent.

- The management team meets regularly with agendered meetings and formal notes.

- The management team reviews its plans regularly and audits performance.

- Appraisal of staff performance is part of the normal organisation, and the clinicians hold regular critical incident sessions to ensure openness and confidence in each other.

- Employment policies are frequently reviewed to keep up with changes in employment law and best management practice.

- Staff views are sought on changes and developments in the practice.

- The practice operates a strong multiprofessional team, with nurse-led clinics.

The staff

- The staff are long-serving and committed with a low turnover and sickness record.

- They are self-motivated and show an enormous amount of initiative.

- They are drawn from the local community and therefore have a good understanding of the community the practice serves.

- They are willing to work flexible hours and overtime.

- They have a good social interaction with each other and the partners.

- They work well as a team and provide a friendly and welcoming atmosphere for patients, locums and other visitors.

- They have good interpersonal skills and handle difficult patients well.

- They contribute to the smooth running of the practice by offering ideas and solutions to problems.

- They give support and encouragement to newcomers.

- Some are ambitious to move into supervisory and management posts and/or want to be appropriately trained and developed for the job.

- They are open-minded towards change and have the capacity to acquire new skills.

The structures and environment

- The premises, both the exterior and interior, have had investment and are well-maintained, showing that patients, partners and staff are valued.

- There are good facilities, such as a pram shelter, disabled access, a staff room, security buttons in the surgeries and reception, clean curtains and carpets.

- The equipment is modern and well-maintained.

- The examination couches have steps up for older and infirm patients and to prevent backache for clinicians.

- The record storage is accessible and easy to use without files dropping on to staff or breaking fingernails.

- The clinical equipment for the doctor on call, in the surgeries and treatment room are regularly checked.

Appendix C
Management tips

1   **Tackle issues immediately.** Inappropriate behaviour needs to be tackled immediately. Not confronting such behaviour at the time, or soon afterwards, fosters resentment on one side and encourages ignorance on the other.

2   **Ask why, and then why again.** Make it a habit to always test assumptions and solutions rigorously to ensure that they are based on clarity and logic, can be justified and solve the problem. If this testing becomes part of your management style, people will expect it and will not take offence, rather they will see it as an essential part of your management of the practice.

3   **Refer staff to the person they are complaining about.** You need to be sure that you are not being manipulated or used as a 'dumping' ground for other peoples' grievances.

4   **Empathise.** Say to yourself 'In this situation, if I was that person, I would feel...'

5   **Support the managers in the practice.** Make it clear that they are managing on your behalf and with your authority.

6   **Model good practice from your clinical experience.** You manage patients and illness everyday, co-ordinate their care, delegate as appropriate, follow-up and monitor results,

and confront poor clinical performance. These skills are transferable to the management of the practice.

7   **Assume the best of motives in others, not the worst**. Let yourself be proved wrong rather than the opposite.

Index